The Second Half of Your Life

Jill Shaw Ruddock

Vermilion

To my husband, Paul, and my daughters, Sophie and Isabella, who have helped make both halves of my life better than I could have ever wished for.

1 3 5 7 9 10 8 6 4 2

This edition published 2011
First published in 2011 by Vermilion, an imprint of Ebury Publishing
A Random House Group company

The Random House Group Limited Reg. No. 954009

Addresses for companies within the Random House Group can be found at www.randomhouse.co.uk

A CIP catalogue record for this book is available from the British Library. The Random House Group Limited supports The Forest Stewardship Council (FSC), the leading international forest certification organisation. All our titles that are printed on Greenpeace-approved FSC-certified paper carry the FSC logo. Our paper procurement policy can be found at www.rbooks.co.uk/environment

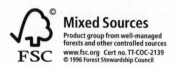

Mixed Sources
Product group from well-managed
forests and other controlled sources
www.fsc.org Cert no. TT-COC-2139
© 1996 Forest Stewardship Council

Printed and bound in Great Britain by Clays Ltd, St Ives PLC

ISBN 9780091939496

To buy books by your favourite authors and register for offers visit www.rbooks.co.uk

Author photograph on cover © Jon Enoch
Author photograph on page 303 © Isabella Shaw Ruddock

Acknowledgements

I n January 2009, when my idea to write *The Second Half of Your Life* transformed from *want* and *would like* to *have* and *need to*, I thought the next couple of years of my life would be spent alone with my thoughts, sitting in front of a computer. As I sat down to write this acknowledgement page, I realised that far from narrowing my world, this experience has actually broadened it and brought me into contact with so many new people, thoughts and ideas. In grabbing for an opportunity that, in the beginning, did not seem possible, the realisation that we can make anything happen in this part of our life became my reality. For two years I lived my life by what I believe are the secrets to successful ageing: exercising, staying connected to family and friends, eating a healthy diet and making passion my purpose every day.

The very writing of this book has done for me exactly what I am advocating for every woman in the decades following menopause – to create opportunities and be brave enough to attempt things that might not work. I set out to write a book that would change the lives of older women, and quite by accident, it changed my life. The huge bonus is that this change was completely unexpected.

I first want to thank my friend Karen Doherty, who introduced me to her fabulous agents Caroline Michel and Robert Caskie from PFD, who believed in this book from the beginning and made a few miracles happen. A special thank you to Fiona MacIntyre, Miranda West, Susanna Abbott and the team at Ebury Publishing for supporting this book the way they did.

Next, a very special thank you to my Kitchen Round Table group, who I depended on more and more as I got closer to publication: Ingrid Jacobson Pinter, Julie Higgins, Libby Pierpont Engstrom, Marsha Lee, Norma Miller, Deborah David, Nancy Casserley, Helen Bromovsky, Hilary Williams, Judy Bollinger, Diana Godding, Louise Bhattacharjee, Penny Mallinson, Catherine Faulks, Nicola Reed, Marianne de Giorgio, Veronica Berman and Stephanie Johannson.

I also want to thank Marie Claire Agnew, Simon Pummell, Veronica and Sebastian Faulks, Sophie Ruddock, Judy Kark, Judy Dewinter, Gwen Snider, Felice Shapiro, Julie Horowitz, Ron Butler, Georgia Newcomb, Greg Johnson, Alfie and Dana Himmelrich, Barbara and Sam Himmelrich, Deborah Kent, Karen Gutman, Marla Rubin, Megan Patel, Annita Bennett, Ellen Miller Gavin, Andrea Sullivan, John and Carolyn Warren, Hollis Rafkin Sax, Susan Whiddington, Jane Horvitz, Barbara and Joe Vittoria, Deborah Kent, Michelle Yang, Noelle Doumar, Heather Acton, Amanda Sater, Peggy Post, Letta Showering, Richard Sharp, Nicolette Kirky, Kate Grussing and Debbie Burston for their contributions to the editorial content of this book. Special thanks to Michael Gutman, Stuart Gillies and Pan Kongsrivilai. I also want to thank Ed Victor, who came up with the title for my book, Claire Alexander, who has been a support to me throughout this process, Rachel Johnson, who published my first article on menopause, David Higgins, founder of Ten Pilates, who kept my body strong, and my new Pilates friends who kept my spirit robust over the past two years: Beverly, Gerry, Emma, Jane and Mina.

When it came to finance, I had some of the best brains in business advising me, and I would like to thank my husband Paul, Bill Bollinger, Jeff Berman, Jerker Johansson, Ben Sax and Christopher Godding. A special thanks to family law solicitors Catherine Bedford and Jeremy Levinson, who guided me through the divorce and separation chapter, David Willetts MP, Minister of State for Universities and Science, Guy Levin, political adviser to the Treasury, who patiently explained the changing pension system, and Dr Marion Gluck and Dr Julie T. Hunter, who worked with me in understanding menopause and hormone replacement therapies.

I would like to thank all the wonderful women who appeared in the promotional film that accompanied the launch of this book: Dame Joan Bakewell, Lynda Bellingham, Tara Gandhi Bhattacharjee, Beth Neilsen Chapman, Susan Hampshire, Sheila Hancock, Kathy Lette, Phyllida Lloyd, Susie Orbach and Mary Wilson, and in particular, I would like to thank Ruby Wax, who has helped me in so many ways throughout the writing of this book and from the very beginning.

I also want to thank all the women who provided their thoughts that appear in Chapter 16. Of course, I could never have convinced many of these gifted and brilliant women to participate without the help of Melanie Hall, Eleanor O'Keefe, John Gordon, Susan Whiddington Margy Kinmonth, Vin Bhattacharjee, Jason Wright, Paula Ridley, Neil Constable, Diana Philips, Matthew Byam Shaw, Hilary Williams, Claire Wilcox and John Williams.

Finally, I would like to thank my husband Paul and my daughters Sophie and Isabella, who have been an incredible support to me throughout this entire process and believed that I could complete the marathon of writing a book and having it published. Sadly, they now know more about hormones and menopause than they ever should at this point in their lives.

Moving forward

'There are people who put their dreams in a little box and say, "Yes, I've got dreams. Of course I've got dreams." They put the box away and bring it out once in a while to look at it and yes, they are still there.'

Erma Bombeck, author

I started writing *The Second Half of Your Life* in response to my own personal circumstances. It evolved and grew into a much bigger book. It began when I was 48 years old and almost through menopause before I realised there was a biological reason why the previous four years of my life were spent wondering who this new person was living in my body. I had suffered and felt very alone.

I never put menopause on my radar screen. I thought it was something that only happened to old people and I was *definitely* not old. In fact, I was still wondering if there was time to have another baby. Every time I missed a period, I would secretly hope there was going to be a 'We really weren't trying. It's a miracle this has happened' moment.

I did not understand what was happening to me or what menopause was. It was simply *never* mentioned. My mother spoke to me about becoming a woman and the arrival of my first period, but she forgot to mention how my body would change again later in life. Menopause never came up in conversation. My friends never discussed it. When it was occasionally mentioned, it was discussed as the beginning of the end, complete with hot flushes, night sweats, depression, moodiness and a lack of libido. It was one great concept shrouded in mystery. I mean, who ever thinks about a car crash until you are actually in one?

By the time I finally went to my doctor, complaining of heart palpitations, depression, 75 hot flushes a day and an under-active thyroid – who gains weight like this unless they have a thyroid problem? – I was, according to my doctor, only a few months away from becoming a post-menopausal woman – a label I would wear for the rest of my life. I needed to get wise quickly!

First, I called a close friend who was 55. I was sure she must know something about this. I asked her to tell me everything she knew about menopause. She said, 'No, I haven't been through the change yet, but I definitely am getting hot flushes.' That conversation hit me like a ton of bricks.

Was I the only 40-something woman in the world who was having internally charged electricity surges, suffering from insomnia and heart palpitations, and finding it necessary to carry around baby powder and three T-shirts to get through the day?

Off to the bookshop I went. There were excellent and comprehensive books ready to answer all my medical questions about the years leading up to menopause; books on how to beat menopause naturally and even how to stay beautiful *in spite* of menopause. There were books on life lessons to be learned and how to give our spirit a make-over when we turn 50. There were so many books about turning 50. Why was 50 such a magical number? What about all the women who were over 50, 60 or 70 years old?

I was just a few months away from becoming a post-meno-pausal woman, and I needed some answers: how to begin to fix the things that were driving me crazy, how to give my life more meaning and overcome the feeling that the best years of my life were behind me? I couldn't find a book that started a dialogue in order for women to openly discuss all aspects of life during and after menopause – a practical 'hands-on' book that didn't just ask the questions women think and worry about, but helped women effectively navigate the obstacles that we will inevitably face during this stage of our lives. Where was the book that offered practical solutions to prepare for the years ahead and guidance about what we care about *after* menopause – in other words, the rest of our lives?

Was my life over as I knew it? Was it a downward spiral from now on? Was I going to become old overnight? Was I going to turn into my mother? I could not work out if I was supposed to be in denial or simply not talk about it. Is menopause supposed to be a secret? Gradually, the idea of writing a book started to germinate. Menopause would be the marker, not the subject. Why?

> Because after we have been through menopause, we are not just the same, only older. Menopause is a rite of passage because it *does* change you, both physically and mentally.

As I got deeper into writing this book, I realised that the changes that occur around menopause encompassed both body and mind. Our brains are no longer fuelled with the hormones that kept us hyper-focused on making babies, raising children and daydreaming about winning a prize in the 'Best Family of the Year' competition. There is a new, hormonally induced desire to finally put our needs first, cultivate dormant passions and reconnect with the world in a different way.

Searching for answers

In the process of writing this book, I spoke with friends, friends of friends, complete strangers, doctors, psychologists, sociologists, solicitors, scientists and health specialists, and attended several conferences. I interviewed over 200 women, each of whom generously shared their own story and ideas about what was helping them to make the changes they needed to make – as well as those things that were standing in the way.

I also assembled a group of 18 conscientious and intelligent women who met regularly. I refer to them as my 'Kitchen Round Table' group. They challenged, argued, cajoled and ultimately guided me to write *The Second Half of Your Life*, and to make it as relevant and important to as many women as possible.

Finally, I sought out visible and influential women who are redefining what it means to grow older and asked each of them to answer the question, 'What advice would you give other women to make the second half of their life the best half?' The answers are fascinating and varied. These quotes make up the bulk of Chapter 16.

It became clear there was another story to be told. The interviews that would form the backbone of this book revealed that most women believed the years after menopause were a time of renewed possibilities, which brought a willingness to push forward with new purpose. However, with new possibilities comes uncertainty.

Today most women share an overriding concern about the quality of life they will lead in the decades following menopause. They know their life expectancy is increasing with every passing year and are searching for answers as to the best way to live the rest of their lives. This searching has created confusion and a desire for answers. One woman said, 'Yes, I know I have lived long enough to know what I want, but I am just not sure how to get what I need. My goals have changed and I am not sure how to get there.'

I have written this book with the belief that it is *how* we choose to embrace this part of our lives that will make the biggest difference to the way we live. Is the glass half-empty or half-full? I hadn't found a book that spoke to me, so I set out to write one. This was clearly a book that needed to be written, and a book that women needed to read.

Could menopause and the second half of our lives be something we might look forward to, rather than dread? Could there be better ways to cope during the years of hormonal havoc before coming out the other side? Nobody seemed to be talking or writing about the menopause and the decades after as a new beginning – a chance to reinvigorate and nurture the best in ourselves, to right some wrongs and become more than the sum of our parts.

It is my hope that menopause will no longer be the unmentionable but an open, accepted and expected part of life's journey to be celebrated and spoken about freely, without embarrassment. Could we dare to dream that the women reading this book now will be openly discussing the joys of post-menopausal life with our peri-menopausal daughters in 20 or 30 years' time?

If the shoe fits, wear it

Menopause is a time in a woman's life when she can pause, prioritise and push towards a new purpose. We now have a renewed drive to achieve some of the goals and dreams we set for ourselves. There is no 'one size fits all' approach to living the second half of our lives; our goals and the scope of change will be different for us all.

Some women will never have had children and possibly have some regrets. Others will still have young children, while others may be excited when their youngest finally leaves home and they have time and space to rediscover themselves. In the same way that some women have horrible PMT (Premenstrual Syndrome) and others don't notice that their periods are coming, some women hardly experience any menopausal symptoms, while for others they can be debilitating.

Among the women I interviewed, there were two attitudes to successful ageing they agreed on: first, preparation and laying a solid foundation for the years ahead was the most important factor in how happily one lives the rest of life, and second, it is never too late to begin again and make the changes that need to be made.

It is how you decide to live the rest of your life that will make the biggest difference to how you grow older: how you find purpose, cultivate a passion, what foods you eat, how much you exercise and how you stay connected to family, friends and your community. I am hopeful you will make these principles, which form the core of my new 'five-a-day', part of your daily life.

I've had my share of life challenges. While running a division of a public investment bank, I balanced my children, my career, my husband, my home and my friends in what often seemed to be a frenetic juggling act. Then, in 1999, I made a big life change. The firm for whom I worked was purchased, and I took the decision to leave. I had two young daughters and no clear idea of what would come next. I *hoped* I was making the right decision, and it turned out I was. This decision completely transformed my life.

I rediscovered my greatest life passion, the theatre, and became involved with the Donmar Warehouse and the Mousetrap Theatre Projects, raising awareness, building community and much-needed funding. I used many of the skills I learned in my years in the City and applied them to an area of my life I care deeply about.

Choice and change

I have written *The Second Half of Your Life* with the belief that every challenge we face is an opportunity to solve a problem. Whoever you are at this very moment, you have a choice. You can be a victim or a champion of change. What you can't be is complacent; standing still is not an option. In the film *Annie Hall,* Woody Allen said, 'Relationships are like sharks. Once they stop moving forward they die.' Getting older is the same: you *have* to keep moving, mentally, physically and spiritually.

You already have everything you will ever need to get started and build on the life you want for yourself. Menopause is a gift. It may not be that blue Tiffany box you always dreamt of, but it is a gift. Using that gift will be empowering and give you the mental and physical strength to be whoever you want to be.

The Second Half of Your Life will not only ask and answer the questions we think and worry about, but also provide practical advice, guidance and structure to make the second half the *best* half.

Shall we begin?

Jill Shaw Ruddock
London, 2010

CHAPTER ONE

Surviving or thriving
For once it really
is about you

'Don't say you don't have enough time. You have exactly the same number of hours in a day that were given to Helen Keller, Pasteur, Michelangelo, Mother Teresa, Leonardo da Vinci, Thomas Jefferson and Albert Einstein.'

H. Jackson Brown, Jr, author

During the first half of life, many of us had a life plan waiting. It was as if we were handed a script and all we had to do was follow it. The script read like this: go to school, go to university, find a job, earn a living, meet a guy, fall in love, plan a wedding, have babies, get your figure back, have more babies, try to get your figure back again, look after the family, cook dinner, do the food shopping, clean the house, pay the bills, go to work, organise repairmen, exercise, make a house a home, meet with teachers, make sure the kids have clothes and shoes that fit, book appointments, schedule activities, coordinate everyone's social lives, plan and book family holidays, make time to talk and listen, ensure you are there (and in the front row) for every school play, every recital, every sports day, sporting event, graduation ceremony and anything else that really matters. You pack up your last child for college ... and then what?

Has anyone been given the script for the second half of life? Most women I know are just not sure how they are supposed to live for the next 30 or 40 years. With a bit of planning, the second half can be just as stimulating and exciting as the first. We know what we like and don't like. We have the accumulated wisdom of all our years, and finally have more of that precious commodity – time – to look after ourselves and do some of the things we always wanted to do.

I know women in their early 60s who look at each passing day as being one step closer to death. I also know women in their 80s who can't wait for the next day. Broadcaster and author Dame Joan Bakewell, now 77, believes her insatiable curiosity and zest is because she is 'greedy, greedy for life'. Creating a framework so we wake up each day with the optimism and vitality to make our lives meaningful and exciting is what each of us needs to ensure we live the life we want.

The power of hormones

Throughout our 20s, 30s and early 40s, our brains relied on heavy supplies of oestrogen (and a few other hormones too), which provided us with a natural mothering instinct, the ability to closely track the emotions of others, and the determination to keep the peace. To transition into marriage and then motherhood, we needed to kiss self-absorption goodbye and make the maximum investment in what our bodies have been doing for hundreds of thousands of years – preparing ourselves for the continuation of the species.

Most women spend the first half of their adult lives trying to please everyone else and putting their own needs last, behind those of their husband, children, parents, friends, colleagues, bosses and repairmen. We do this in order to provide a secure environment in which to raise a family.

Hormones influence our thoughts, feelings and moods. Dr Louann Brizendine, a neuro-psychiatrist and author of the remarkable book *The Female Brain*, states, 'Hormones determine what the female brain is interested in doing ... A post-menopausal woman, not having the fuel of oestrogen, is less concerned with the nuances of emotion and keeping the peace. The mommy brain circuits are finally free to be applied to new ambitions, new thoughts, new ideas. The mommy brain has started to unplug.'

> Giving birth to yourself will surprise, even shock, the people closest to you. The five 'S's – supporting, sublimating, safeguarding, sheltering and shielding – will be replaced with altogether different ones: social life, serious exercise, self-confidence, self-discovery and security.

With this change comes a new sense of stability, creative energy and clarity of vision that helps bring into focus what we need to do to create a happier and more fulfilled second half of life.

Menopause is often referred to as 'the change'. Another word for change is 'transform'. The physical and emotional changes that women go through during peri-menopause – the two-to-nine-year phase leading up to the cessation of periods – give menopause a bad name. Peri-menopause is the time during which our bodies begin to deplete themselves of oestrogen, progesterone and even the male hormone testosterone, producing a series of symptoms that make life feel very challenging.

These symptoms are just signposts to the new road ahead. You are leaving behind a woman who can give birth, but are welcoming a woman who can give birth to herself. The best part of all is that it actually becomes easier to make the kind of changes you have only dreamt of making once you have been through menopause. It is leaving the best for last, and it's definitely worth the wait.

A reawakening

Many women I interviewed believe that the years after menopause have been the best years of their lives. They have felt a 'new confidence sneaking up on them' and want to 'embrace new challenges'. They finally 'feel awake again after so many years of semi-consciousness'. Many women are surprised by the changes. For example, one woman wondered how this new person was able to take over her mind and body. Another asked where the woman had gone who had spent years trying to fix and help those around her.

No one will be more surprised than your family, who may be bewildered by the change in you. When the 'you' they've known for the past 20 years doesn't turn up to cook supper with a smile every evening, they may suspect a nervous breakdown or worry that you are on the verge of filing for divorce from the entire family.

Once you can no longer create biological life, fertility is expressed in a different form – through the creation of new thoughts, purpose and rediscovery. If you haven't quite gone the distance yet and are still in the throes of your peri-menopausal years, your reaction to this next comment will probably range from 'What planet is she on?' to 'If I could run from myself, I would!' But here it is: *Nature did women the biggest favour by designing us to go through menopause.*

Now that you have been through menopause, you will have changed in more ways than one. Menopause will not only alter your hormonal balance, but the way your brain works and the way you look at the world. When the hormones that have made your life hell rebalance again, you will be able to prioritise in a way that will allow you to flourish and blossom. In fact, the hormonally induced transformation of the female brain will alter the way you think and look at the world. It may take some time to recognise and interpret the new messages your brain is sending, but it's definitely talking to you, and you need to start listening. This is change at the deepest level.

A time to re-evaluate

Just around the time women stop getting periods, we start to re-evaluate what matters and wonder if there is something more important out there – something different from the way we have defined our adult lives over the past 30 years. Unlike the men in our lives, who are more prone to a mid-life crisis, we are going through a mid-life re-evaluation. Thoughts such as 'Now is my time', 'It's my turn', or 'There's no time like the present' begin to infiltrate our consciousness, while the voices of self-doubt that prevented us from moving forward in the past become a little quieter. We consciously begin to re-evaluate what matters – and, through this, a new list of priorities is developed.

In Anne Tyler's book *Back When We Were Grownups*, the 53-year-old heroine Rebecca Davitch suddenly realises that she has no idea who she is. In the middle of a boisterous family gathering, she comes to the stark conclusion that she had 'turned into the wrong person'. Have you ever felt like this? You may find in the second half of your life you are breaking the habits of a lifetime in order to become the person you believe you were meant to be, and live a life that is finally about developing the best in *you*.

What's your attitude?

Almost a third of the women I interviewed were unhappy or dissatisfied with their lives because they could not accept getting older – hating every new wrinkle and every tell-tale sign of ageing. The process of ageing has left them depressed, it has affected their marriages, work, family life and the way they view themselves and the world around them.

Many women said they thought it would be all right to slow down both physically and mentally in the second half of their life; however, this type of thinking will set you on the path towards isolation, depression, idleness and debilitating illnesses.

If this sounds like you, you need to start thinking about your Attitude (with a capital 'A'). My mother wanted to be old – and she *was* old by the time she was 60. She stopped exercising, isolated herself from her friends, and watched her body start to fall apart. There is nothing that will make you feel and behave old more quickly than living in a body that has stopped functioning the way it should. By ensuring you have a body that continues to do what it was designed for – walk, run and move – you are giving yourself a true chance of healthy ageing. Many hundreds of thousands of years ago, immobility would have meant instant death because we would have been hunted and killed. It's not so different today. We may no longer be threatened by wild animals, but a lack of mobility leads to the death of independence, health and emotional well-being.

Some women believe they must simply accept the fact that they will get fatter, weaker, lonelier and more crotchety with every passing year. There is almost a passive acceptance that they will be too old to worry about what they look and feel like, and what they still need to accomplish.

Everyone's mindset is different, as are the obstacles and bumps along the way through the second half of life. One aspect of successful ageing that is not up for debate is that the happiest and most vibrant women look after both their emotional and physical health daily. They stay connected to family and friends, exercise and eat a healthy diet, have a passion, and have a purpose that gives clarity and motivation to their life. I call these ingredients my 'five-a-day', and I examine them in more detail later on.

Getting back on the right path

If you have travelled off the path to who you thought you would and *could* be, I am confident that you can and will find your way back again. In fact, you have already taken the first step by reading this book. Most women are complete naturals at making these kinds of changes. Remember, you had to evolve and change in different ways as you moved through your 30s and 40s – juggling the roles of wife, mother, career woman, life and activity coordinator. The second half of your life will be no different. If you don't make changes, you will be fighting an uphill battle to live the life you want.

Up until now, you will have established habits that will be difficult to break. You have nurtured these habits, and they are second nature to you – like a comfortable old pair of shoes with holes which should have been thrown away years ago. Change requires reflection and soul-searching. However, your post-menopausal brain will be beckoning you to put yourself first and become the person you want to be. You simply have to listen – and act.

> It takes strength, awareness, knowledge and commitment to be able to change what is not working. It also requires a willingness to take risks. Many women find it hard to take those first steps for fear of failing. Focusing on the here and now, on what *is* working, and celebrating your successes, one by one, is a good way to start.

Ageing is not a matter of luck

We will each struggle with different parts of ageing. Our skin will wrinkle, our hair will go grey, our bones will become more brittle, close friends will die or move away, and there will be illnesses to battle – our own or those of people we love. Chances are we will live alone for at least some of our adult life, through death or divorce, and money will probably become more and more of an issue. We will miss the everyday life we had with our children.

If you have been unhappy or just not sure who you are any more, now is your time. Only you can decide when and how to focus your energy on changing the parts of your life that are not working. There is choice in all of this. You have several decades left to create, discover, contribute and take on new challenges. It is a great time for rediscovery, hope and new momentum. *We have to age, but we do not have to grow old.*

Although the process of ageing is inevitable, *how* we grow older is something we can control. I am all for accepting what we cannot change. However, acceptance without the desire or the will to change some of the things we don't like about ourselves – the things that we *have* the power to change – means that we have willingly decided to give up living the life we have come to value. Believing that ageing is a matter of luck or about the result of the cards you have been handed in life is not what successful ageing today is all about.

Now is your time

While every woman will be affected differently in the years that follow menopause, 'the change' will propel you forward and help you focus and prioritise on what is important to you now and in the second half of your adult life.

In her book *The Wisdom of Menopause,* Christiane Northrup refers to menopause as a time of confidence – the confidence to begin tomorrow and stay committed to making the changes you need to make to give more meaning to your life. You need to take stock. You need to ask yourself, 'What do *you* want?' After years of sweeping under the carpet your own desires, wishes and dreams in favour of the greater good of your family, it is time for you to use the years of accumulated wisdom to take a second bite of the apple – or even get rid of that rotten apple you've chosen. This is your opportunity to give yourself a second chance – the chance to live the second half of your life as the person you want to be.

How are you going to have the life you want for the rest of

your life? By creating opportunities to find the best in your-self – whether it is going back to fulfil a childhood dream or giving time to a cause that you have always been passionate about – is a good place to start. Growing older, making peace with what you cannot change, rediscovering your strengths, and sharing your gifts with your family, friends and community will not only keep you connected, but also give you new confidence to have the time of your life.

> ❝ Age is the acceptance of a term of years. But maturity is the glory of years. ❞
>
> *Martha Graham, American dancer and choreographer*

We are all living longer. According to Professor Sarah Harper, director of the Oxford Institute of Ageing, 'My mother's life expectancy at my age was her mid-70s; mine is 96! That is two decades more of life in one generation. Every hour we live adds five minutes to our life expectancy.'

It isn't the *number* of years we have left that matter most; it's how we live those years. There are many things that can make you feel 'old' overnight: a failed marriage, depleted bank accounts due to divorce or poor investments, serious illness, irrevocable bodily change, being alone, having no purpose and children leaving home. You may also be coping with ageing parents, fluctuating hormones and the symptoms of ageing, a relationship that has changed or ended, younger children from a second marriage ... all of which need time, energy and money – commodities that may be in short supply.

You may have reached a point where you simply can't work out how to give your life more meaning. The women who most successfully negotiate this change are those who look at their lives with optimism and make positive choices to create what they want from their lives. They realise they have the whole of the second half of their life to complete what they didn't do in the first half. Menopause brings on a change in perspective that fires you in different directions.

What is *your* perfect state of being? Do you know what you would like to change if you could? How you decide to tackle your life 'to-do' list has broad-reaching implications that will determine whether you will thrive or simply survive the next 30 or 40 years of your life. Getting older really can mean getting better. Meeting the challenges you are currently facing head-on is one of the best ways to get through to the other side feeling happier and more successful. It is important to assess what would make a difference in your life. As the personal development guru Dale Carnegie once said, 'Success is getting what you want; happiness is wanting what you get.'

Playing your cards right

If the ultimate goal in the 'big game of life' is to have health, a cohesive family, happiness, a circle of friends on whom you can rely, ease with who you are, and good mental and physical strength, now is the time not only to join the game, but to know what rules will work for you. This is your time to prioritise, be productive, stay active and show the people you love that they are important to you.

Along the way, things break and need to be mended. In fact, this is the time to make sure you fix the parts that can be fixed and live life to the fullest. You cannot rest on your laurels, even if you are 90 years old.

Your new 'five-a-day'

There is little doubt that the obligatory five servings of fruit and vegetables every day form the basis of a healthy diet and good health. However, your *new* five-a-day will give you a new script about how best to reinvigorate yourself. It will help you to fix the things that make you feel less than you are and help to overcome the feelings that the best years of your life are behind you. Incorporating your new five-a-day into your daily life will help make the second half of your life not only good years, but the *best* years of your life.

1. **Stay connected to family and friends:** Figure out how to be helpful to the people who matter most to you. Make socialising your second job. When you say, 'I love you', mean it and say it often. Don't let a little dispute harm a great friendship, so when you make a mistake take immediate steps to correct it. Being isolated may cause you to worry more, as you have no one to share problems with. 'A problem shared is a problem halved.'

2. **Cultivate a passion:** Explore and find the things that bring you joy. Read the books you always wanted to, join or start a book or theatre group, learn a language and then travel to that country, take tennis or golf lessons and play for your local club, learn how to play bridge, join your local choir, take a gardening course, make jewellery or play competitive ping-pong. New activities fire up your brain. Most activities that create new connections, meaning and friendships in this part of our life cost very little money or none at all.

3. **Find a purpose greater than yourself:** Dedicate part of every day to something you are committed to and truly care about. Give your time and energy to help others in any way you can. Get involved with a cause or a charity that matters to you: the arts, local politics, sports, a hospital, school or simply helping an elderly neighbour. Finding purpose can involve going back to college to fulfil a childhood dream or starting the business you always wanted. Look beyond yourself and your immediate world. If you live with purpose, you will live a life that not only gives meaning to those around you, but to yourself as well.

4. **Exercise almost every day of the week:** This will change how you age, feel about yourself and the world around you. The key to exercise (and getting back on the wagon, should you

fall off) is to find an exercise routine you love doing. Whether it is Pilates, spinning, playing tennis or golf, ballroom or salsa dancing, find a class and get moving.   Regular exercise and connecting with your body for at least 30 minutes a day, six days a week, will give you increased vitality, the chance to feel 10 to 30 years younger than your chronological age, while improving your self-esteem, vitality, and how you feel about yourself.

5. **Eat well:** This does not involve a magical mystery tour of supermarkets, health food stores and other specialty shops. Eat primarily foods that come from the ground (fresh fruits and vegetables) good carbohydrates (wholewheat breads, brown rice and legumes) and for your protein eat lean poultry and fish. Stay away from junk food, processed foods and fizzy drinks. By giving your body many of the essential nutrients it needs through the foods you eat, you are giving yourself the best chance to fight disease and avoid other major health problems.

It is finally your time to rediscover the best in yourself, reconnect with the world and make a difference. The choices you make will impact on how you live the second half of your life. This time, it really is about *you*. The great news is that you already have everything you will ever need to get started and build the life you want for yourself.

You have now officially transitioned from your reproductive years to your self-productive years.

CHAPTER TWO

The menopause masterclass

'You must be the change you want to see in the world.'

Mahatma Gandhi

You know the joke about nothing being certain in life except death and taxes? Well, menopause fits into that category too. If you are a woman and you live long enough, you are definitely going to go through menopause. The only questions that are debatable are the number of symptoms you will have, how long the whole process will take and the degree to which you will be affected by 'the change'. Menopause is commonly referred to as 'the change' for good reason: it can change a sweet-tempered lady into an explosive, moody and ill-tempered shrew. Menopause can give the term 'living on the edge' a whole new meaning. For some women, going through menopause is like having PMT every day of the month, but with symptoms that are 10 times worse.

Menopause is all about changing hormones. Most of us have experienced hormonal hell at some point in our lives. Whether you were aware of it at the time or not, you encountered it head on when you went through puberty, during your monthly cycles, when you were trying to get pregnant, once you got pregnant, if you miscarried, after you gave birth, while you nursed your baby or struggled with post-partum depression. The two to six years leading up to menopause, our peri-menopausal years, can feel like a full-blown mugging of our hormones, except you can't file a police report and you won't get much sympathy from anyone who has not been through it.

Menopause separates the time in our lives when we were fertile from the final cycle of our lives, when our ovaries stop producing eggs and our periods stop. It is not a deficiency, not a disease and not an embarrassing problem. It is the end of a woman's reproductive years and a natural part of a woman's life. Although the average age of menopause is 51.4 years in the West, natural menopause can occur any time between the ages of 40 and 58.

Natural menopause can be broken down into three phases, the first two phases take place during peri-menopause, also known as pre-menopause; the last phase is the menopause itself. Technically, the confirmation of menopause is a single-day

Did you know?

- The term menopause was first used in 1879. It comes from the Greek word *mens,* meaning 'monthly', and *pausis*, meaning 'cessation'.

- The British physiologists William Bayliss and Ernest Starling coined the word 'hormone' (from the Greek word *hormon*, meaning 'to spur on') in 1902 to describe secretin, a chemical substance they had discovered.

- Not until around 1925 did modern science discover the human hormonal composition. Only then were they able to differentiate between oestrogen and progesterone.

- The name of the hormone testosterone (T) was coined only in 1935, when Ernest Laqueur isolated it from substances in bull testes.

event because it can only be formally diagnosed exactly a full 12 months after your final period. After this, and for the rest of your life, you are post-menopausal.

You are definitely not alone

Humans are surprisingly unusual when it comes to meno-pause. According to scientists, there are just a few female mammal species that go through menopause: elephants, goril-las, lions and female killer whales. Otherwise, we are on our own. If this distinction feels isolating to you, rather than a cause for celebration, the good news is that about 35 per cent of the female human population is either going through menopause or is post-menopausal. And this number is rising every day.

Although menopause is a universal biological event in a woman's life, women do not readily or openly discuss it. This also makes us feel alone. A close friend of mine told me she has had the same girlfriends for the past 30 or 40 years who were capable of discussing all their deepest secrets and concerns, including sex, relationships and children, but *never* talked about menopause. I don't believe this reticence is the result of not *wanting* to discuss it, but more because we are not sure what is going on and who we are any more.

This also begs the question of the modern male's attitude towards menopause. It is, of course, as varied as the men we know: from intensely curious, interested, questioning and probing to not wanting to know, feeling uncomfortable at the thought of discussing it and hoping it will just disappear.

It is a scary time. Life can seem difficult, unpredictable and feel incredibly unnatural. Do you really want to share the fact you are feeling unbalanced, insecure, anxious, moody and depressed with anyone but your closest confidante? We all have our pride. We want to try and hold on to any shred of normality or sanity we think we might still have.

Symptoms of change

Most women (at least 75 per cent) experience at least a few of the dreaded symptoms during the years that lead up to meno-pause – the peri-menopausal years. Listed below are just some of the symptoms that characterise the hormonal trampoline of your peri-menopausal years.

- **Hot flushes.** More like electricity surges that definitely *do not* light up your life. They are lessened if you cut out alcohol and spicy food, quit smoking and exercise regularly.

- **Sweating.** This can happen day or night, regardless of sub-zero temperatures. Waking up in the middle of the night drenched in sweat is not my definition of fun. Turn off the heat and open the windows, and buy some nightclothes in the new hi-tech fabrics that keep you both cool and dry.

- **Unpredictable periods.** Lighter periods, heavier periods, longer cycles, shorter cycles, you name it. The problem is the unpredictability of it all.

- **Floating anxiety.** Worry can become more exaggerated. Increased fear, anticipating disaster and worrying excessively about health, family, work and money can take over your life. Unfounded fears about taking the train because there might be a terrorist attack, or encountering a natural disaster, such as Hurricane Katrina, can become the cause of many sleepless nights and possibly cancelled travel plans.

- **Panic attacks, depression and heart palpitations.** You may be feeling like a living example of the chicken and egg theory; you aren't sure which came first – the symptoms of depression or your general sense of unhappiness. If you are not sure of the difference between feeling a bit down and being depressed, go to see your doctor. Depression is a disease that needs to be treated. Hot flushes and insomnia, sadly, make this worse.

- **Irritability and moodiness (okay, bitchiness).** Behaviour that used to be within acceptable limits turns into uncontrolled rage over quite unimportant things. It can feel like you are having non-stop PMT. The ability to count to 10 (or 100) will become more useful than it has been since primary school.

- **Trouble sleeping through the night.** Hot flushes, night sweats, the need to urinate at least once (and probably more like three or four times) during the night, anxiety and stress keep you from getting a good night's sleep. You may also find that your brain simply starts sending you a middle-of-the-night wake-up call. Falling back to sleep becomes more difficult.

- **Forgetfulness.** Do I really have the memory of a 90-year-old? One woman confided to me that she was increasingly embarrassed by the fact that she not only forgot things in the short term, but that she sometimes had absolutely no recollection of them. It felt to her as if part of her brain had been erased. Post-it notes can help!

- **Weight gain.** A slower metabolism, a reduction of lean muscle mass (which burns fat) and a redistribution of body fat are common. If you eat the same amount as you did when you were 35, you will need to exercise twice as much and eat half as much just to stay the same weight. Even if you're one of those people who has been blessed with a quick metabolism, you will still have to make some changes to keep the shape you've always had.

- **Itchy, dry and wrinkled skin.** This is a natural part of the ageing process. Our skin not only loses its elasticity, but also its ability to retain moisture. The generation of new skin cells also slows down, which can make skin look dull and lustreless.

- **Dry, thinning and greying hair.** Also a normal part of the ageing process; it is nonetheless alarming to see your once-lustrous locks change colour and texture, and begin to thin and break.

- **Headaches and migraines.** Can be caused by any changes in hormone levels. At their worst, they can feel like someone is drilling holes in your head.

- **Aching joints and sore tendons, muscles and feet.** These are often the product of inactivity combined with normal wear and tear, and can be helped with exercise. If you are always asking your partner for a foot rub, don't necessarily blame your shoes. It might well be another symptom of menopause.

- **Breast tenderness.** This is just a part of the hormonal chaos going on in your body. The good news is that most women don't experience this once menopause has passed.

- **Diminished sex drive.** Otherwise known as 'Where has my libido gone?' You are not alone; this is a common symptom of peri-menopause, along with decreased desire, arousal and sexual satisfaction.

- **Dry vagina.** As if a diminished sex drive wasn't bad enough, the lining of your vagina thins and becomes less moist to the point of arid, making intercourse painful. It can feel a bit like you are losing your virginity every time you have sex. There are solutions. Start by doing Kegels, which strengthen your pelvic floor muscles. An excellent website, if you are not sure of the best way to do them, is www.mayoclinic.com/health/kegel-exercises. More on this later.

- **New allergies.** Changing hormones can bring on a host of new allergies. The most common food and environmental allergens are feathers, pollen, cheese, coffee and shellfish.

- **Insecurities.** Your changing looks, expanding waistline and other parts that just drop overnight, can make you feel self-conscious and depressed, as can the changes that take place in your life. It's not unusual to feel like your world has turned upside-down.

- **Incontinence.** Sneezing, coughing and laughing may be accompanied by involuntary peeing in your pants. You might find that you leak if you don't make regular trips to the loo.

THE MENOPAUSE MASTERCLASS

Kegels are the simplest solution to this, but it's worth noting that slight incontinence is a normal and usually treatable symptom of menopause. Yes, treatable.

- **Urinary tract infections and painful urination.** You are simply more prone to these infections during peri-menopause. It is all part of the hormonal elevator (going down, please!). See your doctor immediately with any symptoms because the infection can spread to your kidneys if left untreated.

- **Feelings of purposelessness and isolation.** The focus of your life changes as you hit the second half. You may need to let go of long-held dreams. You may have to adjust to your children leaving home or the end of your marriage. You may come to the point where you decide that the life you have been living is not the one you want to have for the next 40 years. It's natural to experience emotional turmoil, and that turmoil is heightened by the reduction of hormones in your body. Be aware of this before you both decide to 'throw in the towel' for the wrong reasons.

Three kinds of menopause

Natural menopause usually takes place some time between the ages of 40 and 58 in women who have at least one of their two ovaries.

Premature menopause occurs in women under 40. When it occurs naturally, the primary reasons are an autoimmune disorder or genetics (your mother probably went through menopause prematurely).

Artificial or induced menopause affects one out of every four women. It occurs when both ovaries are surgically removed during a hysterectomy, or after chemotherapy or radiation.

Déjà vu

Your years of peri-menopause are a bit like puberty all over again, and you remember how much fun that was? Puberty was a time when we experienced significant body changes that completely preoccupied us. We became more self-absorbed, wondering how to give our lives more meaning. Our relationships changed and became more complex. We experimented, became more independent and began to look outside the family to confirm our identities. Our focus shifted from our immediate family to the wider world.

It was a challenging and confusing, yet dynamic, period in our life, and we emerged with a new awareness and desire to start building independence on the foundations we had laid. Thirty-five years on, you may have a feeling of déjà-vu overcome you as you struggle once again with physical and emotional changes, and look for new ways to give meaning to your life.

When you pause to consider the big changes that have taken place in your life as a woman, it's worth remembering a single word: hormones. Why do you think you woke up one morning at about 12 or 13 years of age to find yourself suddenly interested in boys and actually wondering what it would be like to kiss one? Hormones. What do you think made your biological clock tick so loudly that it became almost deafening? Hormones.

Many of life's key biological stages are influenced and even determined by hormones – as the balance of oestrogen, progesterone and testosterone shifts and then shifts again. It is those same hormones (this time depleted) that are reconfigured during the years leading up to menopause, creating a host of symptoms that let you know your fertile years are nearly over. Without these hormones, you will begin to have renewed clarity and a passion for life. According to Deborah Blum, author of *Sex on the Brain*, 'Hormones profoundly affect our behaviour. Hormones are what make us tick.'

Your transformation

The hormones that govern this mid-life transformation will not only change your body, but your mind and spirit at the deepest level. There has been a lot of research published about the physiological changes that affect women during their post-menopausal years. Just as your body is changing, depleting itself first of progesterone, then testosterone and finally oestrogen (you will find that you start to gain weight by just thinking of eating a piece of lemon tart), your brain is changing too.

It is important to remember that the changes that define menopause are not only physical, but cerebral as well. After going through the first two phases of menopause, when you think you might be losing your mind, you *do* find it again and it is firing on all cylinders. So you just need to make sure you have a good place to drive to.

Am I pregnant?

The change can arrive at any time. When I entered the final year of my peri-menopause as I turned 48, it had not even crossed my mind that menopause could be the reason why I was feeling and thinking the way I was. And, believe me, I was not thinking particularly uplifting and cheery thoughts.

When I finally went to my doctor, a year later, complaining of depression, insomnia, heart palpitations and somewhere between 50 and 75 hot flushes a day, I said to him, 'I am not sure, but could this have anything to do with menopause?' He looked at me and then asked when my last period was. To be perfectly honest, I wasn't certain. Things had become so irregular that I wasn't sure if I would get my period every 21 days or every 60 days. I had simply been relieved that I didn't have to deal with my periods quite so regularly. Little did I know that this was all part of the menopausal journey.

My doctor suggested a blood test to measure the levels of my reproductive hormones, which I recommend you get now so you have a baseline measurement. You may also be offered an ultrasound scan to see how your uterus and ovaries are faring, as well as a bone-density scan to check for any degeneration in the strength of your bones. I had all of these, as well as a full check of my thyroid gland, because I was convinced that an under-active thyroid could be the only reason for my recent, inexplicable weight gain.

Two days later my doctor called to say that he had the results of my blood tests. I immediately asked, 'Am I menopausal?' He said, 'No.' I started to get excited, thinking of names for our next child. 'Am I pregnant?' He said, 'No, you are post-menopausal. There is not even a trace of oestrogen in your blood. I think that some time over the next three months, all of your symptoms will completely disappear.'

Needless to say, I was in shock – but also relieved to know that I wasn't going to feel or act this way for the rest of my life. My peri-menopausal years were almost over, and I was going to come through it very soon. Then, he said something that I will never forget for as long as I live. He asked me if I would like to go on 'the Pill', as some women miss getting their periods and it could help relieve some of the peri-menopausal symptoms. Did I feel I had lost something important to me by not getting a monthly period any more? I can assure you that the thought never crossed my mind – and hasn't in all the years since saying goodbye to this monthly event.

The phases of menopause

There are three very defined phases of menopause, which all together can last for years. In fact, the typical length of the whole transition is five and a half years. You may be one of a relatively small number of women who hardly noticed any changes before the menopause. You are done. Consider yourself lucky. For some women, the symptoms of peri-menopause can last as long as

15 years. Do yourself a favour and do not read this last paragraph to your husband or partner; this is a lose–lose situation!

Phase one: let the games begin

Peri-menopause is a bit like the child's game Chinese whispers. Your brain and your ovaries, which have been communicating extremely well for the past 30-plus years, start speaking in different tongues. Since the beginning of menstruation, the hormones oestrogen and progesterone have complemented each other very nicely. All of a sudden, as your progesterone levels start to drop off a cliff, you become 'oestrogen dominant'. The result? A huge misunderstanding between the brain and the rest of your body, in which all hell breaks loose. Failing to understand what your brain is saying, your body starts to produce more oestrogen, and that creates some of the classic symptoms of peri-menopause.

One of the first signs of peri-menopause for most women is missing a couple of periods – or suddenly experiencing them non-stop. I was always as regular as clockwork, so when I missed a period, I would secretly be thinking of names for my next child. I would convince myself that I was pregnant, and run out to buy several pregnancy tests. I couldn't believe that I was going to be a mother again at 44. Instead, this was the beginning of the end of my fertility, but I didn't know it yet.

Your menstrual cycle can be affected in other ways too. You might, for example, bleed for weeks on end, which could provoke all sorts of anxiety and concern that you might be suffering from a serious illness. Your menstrual cycle may also become shorter, and therefore your periods will occur closer together. This is because your ovaries are starting to tire. They will eventually become exhausted and run out of eggs altogether. If you don't know what's happening, you might think that more frequent periods are a sign of fertility, when what is really happening is that your ovaries are in the first phase of signing off for life. After this, your cycles will become further apart and then stop altogether.

GOOD-BYE PROGESTERONE

During phase one of peri-menopause, progesterone levels drop to almost zero. Progesterone is a hormone produced by the ovaries and in many ways it counterbalances the effects of oestrogen. Progesterone brings about the release of an egg from the ovaries. When an egg is not fertilised, it is progesterone that stimulates the lining to shed, causing a period. Progesterone's main job is to help the body prepare for pregnancy by promoting the survival and development of the embryo and foetus.

Normal levels of progesterone ...

- Increase your metabolic rate so that you burn more calories when you are resting.

- Stabilise blood-sugar levels, which help our bodies use and eliminate fat.

- Help your thyroid hormone, which is your body's energy and heat regulator.

- Encourage deep, restful sleep.

- Reduce stress and depression, and regulate mood swings.

- Bring about a sense of well-being.

- Help your body eliminate excess fluid.

- Build bone tissue.

Not surprisingly, lower levels of progesterone cause a host of symptoms, many of which are linked to weight and energy levels. When your progesterone levels drop during peri-menopause, you can expect bloating, weight gain, insomnia, cramping, mood swings and tender breasts. Lower progesterone levels can also cause other gynaecological problems, such as endometriosis, painful periods, irregular bleeding and fibroids.

CHEERIO TESTOSTERONE

Testosterone isn't just for men. Women also need it. During phase one of peri-menopause, women lose 70 per cent of their testosterone as production from the ovaries and adrenal glands slows dramatically. This hormone affects energy levels, muscle mass, body fat, tolerance for exercise, mood, bone density and stamina. What's more, lower levels can result in a severely decreased sex drive, difficulty in achieving orgasm, weaker and different orgasms, discomfort during intercourse and even headaches. All those classic 'Not tonight – I have a headache' jokes have a medical basis. Now you know why!

Normal levels of testosterone ...

- Build muscle, increase muscle tone and reduce fat deposits in the body.

- Strengthen bones.

- Increase sexual desire.

- Provide a sense of confidence.

- Deliver energy and help you withstand stress.

- Decrease cholesterol levels.

- Relieve joint and muscle pain.

It is during phase one of peri-menopause that you start to feel like you don't live in your own body any more. There have not, to date, been any movies made about this phase of menopause, but if there were, some titles might be: *Invasion of the Body Snatchers*, *Alien*, *Is That Really My Mother?*, *It* Was *a Wonderful Life*, *Big*, *Heat*, or *I'm Complicated*.

Phase two: puberty in reverse

Do you recall when you were a teenager and you would run to the bathroom to check out the new spots on your face?

You couldn't wash your face fast enough because oestrogen levels were rising so fast. Oestrogen is everywhere in your body. Oestrogen is the major hormone responsible for turning a girl into a woman. It helps control menstruation, pregnancy, regulates body temperature, and has a major impact on the entire body.

In phase two of peri-menopause, oestrogen levels start to drop precipitiously – hence puberty in reverse. As in phase one, phase two also occurs before menopause actually occurs. When your body starts to deplete itself of oestrogen, you can experience just a few or the whole range of symptoms, as well as some more serious health problems, such as osteoporosis and hardening of the arteries.

Normal levels of oestrogen regulate ...

- Skin elasticity.

- Menstrual cycle.

- Concentration and memory.

- Lubrication of the vagina.

- Balance and coordination.

- Bone strength and density.

- Health of blood vessels, i.e. cardiovascular functions.

- Depression and anxiety.

- Good balance of blood cholesterols.

PREPARE FOR THE WORST, HOPE FOR THE BEST

It is important for you to be aware of the impact of falling oestrogen levels so you can become emotionally and physically prepared. Hormones rule our life and who we are on any given day. Of course, you may be one of the lucky few who barely suffers at all. However, it is best to prepare for the worst and hope for the best. How we choose to educate ourselves, view our own change and make the necessary lifestyle change in our daily life that will make a difference in how we cope with menopause and the decades that follow. While I was in the middle of peri-menopause I knew I had a great life, a wonderful husband and children I loved. I was even lucky enough to be able to rediscover and channel my passion for the theatre. Yet I felt unhappy in a way that I could not shake. I also had a shorter fuse, which seemed to explode on impact for no rational reason. I couldn't figure it out.

Feeling stressed and unhappy is different from depression. Depression can rear its ugly head, particularly during this time of life. The death of a parent, an unexpected change in your marriage, empty nest syndrome or lack of sleep can all contribute to feeling depressed. Since oestrogen assists in the formation of neurotransmitters such as serotonin, which helps relieve depression and anxiety, the drop in oestrogen production can exacerbate feelings of depression. Many women suddenly develop displaced anxiety and have panic attacks as they head towards the menopause. It is worth noting that the vast majority of these symptoms disappear when you move into your post-menopausal years – the next 30 or 40 years of your life.

Phase three: menopause and post-menopause

It may sound strange, but, technically speaking, menopause is declared 'official' exactly 12 months to the day after your last menstrual cycle. The day after that – and for the rest of your life – you are post-menopausal. As both progesterone and oestrogen have now levelled off at their new lower levels, previous symptoms diminish and you start to get the clarity, balanced perspective, peace of mind, and in many cases the heightened energy which may have been missing for a while. I have to point out that some women continue to experience hot flushes and other symptoms of peri-menopause into their 60s and 70s. This does not mean you are not post-menopausal.

Societal symptoms

The way women experience menopause varies enormously in different parts of the world. How a woman perceives menopause is coloured by her culture and her views on ageing and sexuality. According to the American Society for Reproductive Medicine, 'Stereotypically, Western women face the menopause with dread, fearing the decline of feminine allure so important in a youth-oriented society. In contrast, Asian women, living in a culture that venerates the elderly, welcome this phase and have a lower prevalence of menopausal symptoms.' A new study published in *Climacteric*, the journal of the International Menopause Society, found that British women suffer the worst menopausal symptoms in the world. Researchers found that many of our symptoms directly correlate to how society views older women; in other words, are they revered or do they become invisible with age?

Are Western women really destined to endure years of misery once the transition into menopause begins? By making some relatively small changes to your lifestyle and adopting my new five-a-day (see page 24), you can go a long way towards reducing many of these symptoms. The latest research supports that almost 85 per cent of women find relief through nutritional, dietary and lifestyle changes.

Of your new five-a-day, regular exercise and nutrition are the most important as they will have an impact on the way that every single part of your body functions. We'll look at this in more detail in the next two chapters. However, each of my new five-a-day will play a role in changing the way you feel about yourself and your life, which will have a positive impact on your symptoms and the rest of your life.

Hormone therapy: the great debate

In life, we are constantly evaluating the risks we are willing to take versus the rewards we will reap. For some women, hot flushes, night sweats and vaginal dryness are simply annoying, but for others completely unbearable. Only you and your doctor can assess the best course of action to get you through this time. If your symptoms are overwhelming you, interrupting your sleep, making you depressed, or disrupting your sex life, and hence the functioning of your marriage and your relationship, you may decide you would like to have help by way of either conventional (i.e. synthetic) hormone replacement therapy (HRT) or bio-identical hormone replacement therapy (bHRT). HRT involves replacing the hormones oestrogen, progesterone and testosterone in your body.

Three kinds of hormones

Natural: the ones made by your own body – namely, oestrogen, progesterone and testosterone.

Synthetic: any hormone not produced by the human body.

Bio-identical: synthetic drugs whose chemical structure matches identically hormones produced in the body.

What is natural?

The term 'natural' means something derived from nature. When it comes to hormones, the only kind of natural hormones that exist are those produced by the body. In theory, HRT, which is made from the urine of a pregnant mare, could be considered natural, just as bio-identical hormones derived from plants could also be thought of as natural. However, neither are natural as they are synthesised in a laboratory and are chemicals.

The bottom line is that *all* hormone treatments are synthesised drugs and none of them are completely natural. The same rule applies for bio-identical HRT as it does for conventional/synthetic HRT – take the lowest dose for the shortest amount of time (Women's Health Initiative recommendation). Whichever hormone replacement therapy you choose, you and your doctor should review your treatment every 6–12 months.

The medicalisation of menopause

Hormone treatment for women started at the turn of the 20th century, but really took off in the 1960s when gynaecologist Robert Wilson published a book, *Feminine Forever,* touting the virtues of oestrogen treatment for the older and grumpy wife. His proposition was that oestrogen would bring back the woman who lived to serve her husband. Hormone therapy was hailed as the magic new medicine, and there was a rush by the pharmaceutical companies to produce and market it.

Oestrogen in the form of Premarin was *the* drug of choice (well, almost!) until 1975, when it was linked to a rise in endometrial cancer. Sales plummeted until doctors started to add progestin (similar to progesterone) in the form of Prempro to hormone therapy, which seemed to do the trick. Hormone therapy was believed to decrease the risk of cancer, and women having the combination therapy – which is used today – showed them to have stronger bones and a lower risk of heart disease. Annual prescriptions soared.

In 1991 the US-based Women's Health Initiative (WHI) launched the largest study to date (161,000 post-menopausal women between the ages of 50 to 79) to see if the benefits of HRT outweighed the increased risk of various cancers. This study was stopped in 2002, three years early, as women taking the oestrogen–progestin combination were recognised to be at higher risk of blood clots, heart attacks and breast cancer.

If your symptoms are particularly debilitating, you might be tempted to head straight to your doctor to ask for a prescription for hormone replacement therapy. The treatment drugs are available as tablets, skin patches, gels, nasal sprays, vaginal rings or skin implants. HRT was one of the first options my doctor suggested when my menopause was diagnosed, and it didn't take me long to reject it. I knew of too many women who thought they were getting a magic bullet with HRT, but instead felt like they were going crazy and went on to gain lots of weight.

When HRT first emerged on the scene, the oestrogen used, as it is today, was considered to be natural as it was derived from the urine of pregnant mares hence the name Premarin – *pre*gnant *mare*s' ur*ine*. Many people, including myself when faced with the option of should I or should I not, found this an unsettling thought. Horse oestrogen did not seem natural for women. Perhaps this is the reason why so many women complained of growing to be 'as big as a horse' on this therapy. Another word of caution if you are allergic to horses, you definitely want to choose another treatment.

If you think conventional HRT is the best option for you, take time to talk to your doctor about the side effects, the risks and the options. There are many women who swear by conventional HRT and don't think they could have made it through their perimenopausal years with it. However, many women I interviewed said they felt like 'Jekyll and Hyde' characters, alternately depressed and irritable, when they started HRT. You might think you are giving yourself a new lease of life, but it may not work out that way for you.

Bio-identical hormones

Bio-identical hormones are derived from plant sources, such a soya beans and yams, and have an identical structure to the hormones our bodies produce, hence the term bio-identical. This is not about rubbing wild yams over your body, as Kim Cattrall did in *Sex in the City 3*. Many bio-identical hormones have been created in a laboratory, and some are produced by major pharmaceutical companies and are approved by the

Federal Drug Administration (FDA) in the United States and the Medicines and Healthcare Products Regulatory Agency (MHRA) in the UK. Bio-identical oestrogen products, such as Vagifem, Ovestin, Elleste Solo and Estraderm, as well as bio-identical progesterone products, such as Gestone and Utrogestan, and bio-identical testosterone, Testogel, are all available and manufactured by the major pharmaceutical companies.

Bio-identical HRT differs from conventional HRT in that, as the name suggests, it is identical to the body's hormones. Because it has the same molecular structure, the receptors in our cells utilise them more efficiently and are much less likely to reject them. Bio-identical HRT can also be used more flexibly – in other words, not with a 'one dose fits all' approach. You can be given a customised blend of oestrogen, progesterone and testosterone in doses that are tailored to your individual needs. While many of these drugs are government approved, others are not tested for consistency by any regulatory agencies. Be careful of false claims and buying products on the internet or over the counter.

Suzanne Somers, in her books *Ageless* and *Sexy Years*, is a big advocate of the use of bio-identicals, and believes conventional HRT is dangerous and unnecessary to relieve the symptoms of menopause. 'Made from pregnant mares' urine and pharmaceuticalised in a one pill fits all therapy, HRT has been proven to be harmful to our health.' She may be right about this, but proposing that bio-identicals will keep women feeling young and sexy forever is selling them a false bill of goods.

Having said that, Dr Marion Gluck, co-author of *It Must Be My Hormones: Getting Your Life Back with Bio-Identical Hormone Therapy and Nutrition*, and a pioneer in the use of bio-identical hormones, claims that, 'Bio-identical hormones are a safe alternative to help women get their lives back and feel normal again through menopause and old age. The wonderful thing about these hormones is that the body recognises them as their own. Over the past 15 years, I have found that I can dramatically lower the dosages of hormones I prescribe, with the same effect. It won't keep you looking young but it will help you feel normal again, give you back your energy, and get the balance back in your life.'

Many women assume that bio-identical is a natural, herbal remedy, but it is not. It is a pharmaceutical product that is synthesised from natural ingredients in a series of chemical steps. In other words, the active ingredients are extracted in the lab and bottled.

This same process also applies to 'natural' oestrogen, progesterone and testosterone products sold by pharmaceutical companies or compounding pharmacies, which are often derived from other parts of the wild yam and from soya beans. These are not natural herbal remedies; they are bio-identical hormone replacement therapy – hormones that have been synthesised in the lab. Remember, with all forms of HRT, the recommendation of the Women's Health Initiative is to take the lowest dose for the shortest amount of time. Bio-identical hormones should not be taken indefinitely and should not be viewed as a 21st-century version of the 'fountain of youth'.

Non-HRT options

Many women I know are reluctant to begin taking drugs to control symptoms, even if their symptoms are horrible. Hormone replacement is not the only therapy available to you. Most women who add exercise and a healthy diet to their daily life see a marked improvement in their menopausal symptoms. In fact, there is plenty of research to support this finding. Some have found that homeopathy and acupuncture helped them cope with peri-menopausal symptoms.

I am not here to recommend or warn you against any one treatment, but I would advise you that there are risks involved in any type of hormone replacement therapy. Start with the lowest dose and move up if you aren't feeling any better. Most new research points to negative outcomes in the long term use of any type of hormone treatment, so remember to re-evaluate after six months.

Getting through your menopausal years

Good health and creating a general sense of well-being are key to negotiating the variety of symptoms that can crop up during the years leading to menopause. And because this is the time in your life when things can start to go wrong, it is extremely important to focus on your own health, have regular check-ups and make yourself aware of some of the risks you face.

Improve your knowledge of medical science and make it work for you. The more you educate yourself, the more able you will be to participate actively in your own health. In the Further Reading section (see page 297) I list many reference books and websites that you can use to guide you through your peri-menopausal years. Healthy, strong women don't just survive – they *thrive*. The following tips will help you to do just that.

My top 10 tips

1. **Make sure you schedule an annual appointment** with your GP, gynaecologist, eye doctor, otologist (ear doctor), dermatologist and dentist.

   - *Ask your gynaecologist* for a blood test to analyse your hormone levels. Once you know where you are in your transition to menopause, you can make some decisions about the best way to deal with the symptoms you may be experiencing now, and the way you want to approach your health in future.

   - *Get a bone density scan* (DEXA scan) to find out your risk of osteoporosis (thinning of the bones). Our bones become weaker without oestrogen to protect them, and apart from a proper diet, strength and weight-bearing exercise to keep them strong, you may need some supplementary vitamins (calcium and vitamin D) and low-dose hormone treatment to ensure that they maintain their health. You will also need to focus on a diet that gives you the nutrients your bones need to stay healthy.

• *Get a mammogram* at least once every two years, and request an ultrasound if you have fibroid dense breasts, which often obscures cancer in mammograms. Also remember to examine your breasts at home. Half of all cases of breast cancer occur between the ages of 50 and 69, with 25 per cent occurring over the age of 70. Be vigilant.

• *Look after your skin.* When you check your breasts for lumps, check yourself for any changes on your skin, such as new moles or moles that have changed colour or size, especially if you are fair-skinned.

• *Look after your eyes.* Eye changes are common as a result of lower oestrogen levels. Dry eyes, having difficulty reading and UV damage all come with the territory. Eat lots of vegetables containing vitamin A, and the bright orange and yellow foods that contain carotenoids. Finally, don't forget your sunglasses. Apart from being one of the greatest fashion accessories known to womankind, sunglasses can help to stave off eye disease.

• *Get your hearing checked.* What did you say? Most people experience some degree of hearing loss as they age. Of course, if you were cranking up the stereo to 120 decibels to listen to The Who when you were younger, you probably damaged some of the cells in your inner ear. If you are hard of hearing, there are many more options available today. Many companies now offer 'fully digital programmable hearing aids'. These are like little mini computers you can wear in your ears, capable of monitoring different audiological environments.

2. **Quit smoking.** It exacerbates every symptom of menopause and increases your chances of serious illnesses in the second half of your life.

3. **Get into a good sleep routine that works for you.** Lack of sleep can magnify everything that's negative about your life. It is linked to conditions such as high blood pressure, stroke, diabetes, obesity and alcohol and drug abuse. When we don't get enough sleep we eat more, become tired and irritable, find it difficult to motivate ourselves to exercise and seek out new passions and interests, and also struggle to concentrate. You can encourage good sleep by eating foods rich in the amino acid tryptophan (found in milk, bananas and turkey), and also by developing a good sleep routine – going to bed at a regular time, avoiding falling asleep in front of the television, cutting down on caffeine and reducing your alcohol intake. Keep your bedroom cool at night. Turn off the heat and open your windows.

4. **Include phytoestrogens in your daily diet.** These are a group of chemicals found in plants that can act like the hormone oestrogen. They are particularly useful for menopausal women, not only because they can help to ease symptoms of menopause, but because they can help to protect your bones and lower cholesterol. Soya beans and soy products, such as tofu, are by far the best sources, but other good sources include wholegrains, beans, nuts, seeds, seed oils, berries, fruits, vegetables and roots (see page 95).

> ## Unplugged!
>
> If you struggle to fall asleep, awaken frequently in the night, or feel groggy and under the weather, try this. Every night for the next two weeks, unplug *all* of your electrics (including your toaster, kettle, hairdryer, microwave, Sky box, washing machine and computer), and make sure everyone in the house turns off their mobile phones and any wireless connections for broadband. Turn off *everything*. There is a growing body of evidence to suggest that electro-pollution can damage your health. My husband and I are both sensitive to electro-pollution and making this small change to our lives has led to a big improvement in the way we sleep and feel on every level.

5. **Watch your weight.** Being overweight can play havoc with the hormonal activity in your body, partly because fat cells can manufacture hormones as well as store them, which upsets the balance you're after. Furthermore, being overweight can affect your health on every level and lead to many health problems, including heart disease, stroke and diabetes. Keep an eye on your BMI (body mass index), which will give you an idea whether your weight is right for your height, or whether it is creeping into obesity territory, where your health is at risk.

   To calculate your BMI, measure your height in metres and multiply that figure by itself, then divide it by your weight in kilograms. For example, if you are 1.6 metres tall and weigh 65kg, you would have the following calculation:

   1.6 x 1.6 = 2.56
   65 ÷ 2.56 = 25.39

This means your BMI is 25.

A BMI of 18.5–24.9 is normal; 25–29.9 is overweight; and 30 and above is obese. Of course you can just Google 'calculate my BMI' and 390,000 websites will pop up and do the calculations for you. An easy-to-use site is http://www.nhs.uk/Tools/Pages/Healthyweightcalculator.aspx.

Are you an apple or a pear?

Even more important than your weight is your shape. Apple-shaped women carry weight around their middle, which is considered the unhealthiest place for weight to accumulate. Why? Because this type of fat (known as intra-abdominal fat, or IAF) is closely associated with Type 2 diabetes, as well as an increased risk of female cancers. It's worth pointing out that as oestrogen supplies dwindle, most women do start storing more fat around their abdomen, which makes it increasingly important to keep it off. Pear shapes have a smaller waist than they do hips, and are less likely to suffer from health disorders. A simple way to check this is to measure your waist. In women, apples have a waist circumference of about 90cm (35+ inches).

6. **Work out if your depression is something more than just feeling low.** Depression can become a bigger problem during and after menopause. The loss of a spouse, parents, siblings or close friends becomes more likely during this period. Health and financial worries can increase. You may lose your sex drive. Changes in your physical appearance and the loss of some of the roles that gave your life meaning can all join the list of things you worry about, as can taking on additional responsibility for ageing parents. If symptoms

of lethargy, exhaustion, hopelessness, short temper or lack of motivation occur for longer than two weeks, consult your doctor. Depression is a disease that needs to be treated. Women are twice as vulnerable to depression as men.

7. **Stay connected to others:** family, friends and your community. Take the time to be helpful, show gratitude when someone is kind to you or has gone out of their way to help you, and do not harbour grudges. Create traditions that matter for the people in your life who matter. Forgiveness of others and yourself is important because ultimately the only person you are hurting is yourself. Forgiveness is a simple concept but, as we all know, simple isn't always easy.

8. **Keep your mind active.** Cultivating a passion and having a purpose means you will be surrounding yourself with people who inspire and motivate you. See Chapters 6 and 7 for the best ways to do this.

9. **Exercise regularly.** I can't stress this enough. My own personal experience has shown that this is the single best way to feel great after menopause and live a healthier life. Exercise enhances health on every level, the mind and body connection is not something to be laughed at. We examine in greater detail the benefits of regular exercise in the next chapter.

10. **Look after your heart.** Heart disease is the number one cause of death in post-menopausal women, mainly because the drop in oestrogen and progesterone causes the blood vessels to become less elastic and more constricted. Eat well, exercise regularly, cut down on alcohol and establish a healthy weight to give your heart the best chance of survival. And if you have a family history of heart disease, tell your doctor, who can arrange for tests to gauge how susceptible you are and could become.

These tips will not only increase your odds of achieving a healthy and happy second half of your life, but they will help you to look and feel younger. In contrast to Alexander Pope, I believe that a little knowledge is not a dangerous thing; in fact, it can be empowering. Knowledge gives us choices in the way we lead our lives. Taking the necessary precautions to prevent health problems is more important now, and you need to make this a priority. Along with this, actively seeking a lifestyle that can provide you with the energy, motivation, optimism, strength and vitality you need is essential to make the second half of your life what you want it to be.

Will you be able to make peace with what you can and cannot change? Can you make some small changes so you can create a new equilibrium that will help you achieve your goals during the second half of your life? If you are not sure how to do this, keep reading. If you have the determination to pursue good health, stay close to your family and a few good friends, have a curiosity about the world around you, and the desire to get involved in causes you care about, the best years are yet to come.

CHAPTER THREE
Regular exercise
Emphasis on 'regular'!

'Normal ageing isn't normal. Decay is not biological ageing. Decay comes from giving up on life and failing to engage. Ageing is up to nature, but decay is up to you. Think of exercise as sending a constant grow message to get stronger, more limber and functionally younger.'

Chris Crowley and Henry S. Lodge, Younger Next Year

Anybody who told you that you only need to exercise two or three times a week is either in their 20s or 30s, a man under the age of 50, or someone who hasn't gone through menopause. Six days a week (even God got one day off when creating the universe), 30 minutes a day – four strength and two aerobic sessions – is what is required to look and feel your best in the second half of your life.

Regular exercise will make the biggest difference to your quality of life for the *rest* of your life. This is the 21st-century version of the 'fountain of youth'. Both muscular and aerobic exercise will boost muscle mass and increase your flexibility and metabolism. When you incorporate exercise into your life six days a week, you will be helping yourself to lower your chances of getting type 2 diabetes, high blood pressure, heart disease, some types of cancer and debilitating joint and muscle pain. A sedentary life will put you on the road to early ageing and take away your ability to live the rest of your life with passion and purpose.

A lot of this chapter is about getting started. If your time is at a premium or you lack the inclination to exercise, the thought of four sessions of muscle-strengthening exercise and another two sessions of aerobic exercise every week may be enough to make you flip straight to the next chapter. Please don't. Finding an exercise routine that you actually enjoy will make the biggest difference to how you are able to live the second half of your life.

Human beings were designed to hunt or to be hunted, build shelter, stay warm, plant and harvest food and have children. Basically, our bodies were built to keep moving until we died naturally or were killed. If you think about how hard Neanderthals had to work, it makes sense that our bodies crave a pumping heart and some serious muscle work. Neanderthal women had to build shelters, chop the wood for fires, go hunting for mammoths and sabre-tooth tigers, and then cook them. There was no division of labour. Women joined men in the hunt.

By the time the 20th century rolled around, women were still getting their aerobic workouts doing domestic chores – washing dishes, scrubbing and sweeping floors, raking leaves, flipping beds, beating rugs and washing clothes by hand. Household chores were truly exhausting.

Yet here we are, just over a decade into the 21st century, and we can do virtually everything we need to without leaving the comfort of our La-Z-Boy chairs. We can do our weekly food shop on the internet and have it delivered right to our kitchen; efficient dishwashers and washing machines do much of the cleaning and laundry; our newspapers can be delivered to our computers or iPads each morning; fast food is available on every high street; and if you don't crave something quick at McDonald's, there are ready-made dinners to purchase from Marks & Spencer or Tesco. The reward for all this hard work? A nice glass of cold Sauvignon Blanc and a big bowl of kettle chips while sitting in front of the television to catch up on the news of the day.

When and how do you give your body what it was originally designed to do? As a nation we are living longer due to medical breakthroughs, but our bodies are not keeping up with the number of years we are on this earth. Exercise is absolutely necessary when it comes to menopause and the rest of your life. Without building muscle and aerobic strength, year on year you will become weaker, slower and fatter, and you will be forced to live with pain. Exercise is the only way to combat nature's laws of life, ageing and disease.

> The body is a wasting asset and we all definitely
> have a sell-by date, but we can extend our
> shelf life!

Putting a spring in your step

Modern medical technology will not be able to help you. Yes, people are living longer, but the quality of life in the last 10 or 20 years of our lives basically stinks. The best way to plan for a vibrant future is to incorporate strength training and aerobic exercise into your daily life. Having a body that is ready for action will change how you grow old and how you feel about yourself and the world around you. We all know what old *sounds* like. Listen to your body and get moving.

The end result of keeping fit is that you will manage your stress better, you will feel more energetic and alert, you will lower your risk of many diseases, and you will feel better about yourself and your body. The best part is that you can make it fun, make new friends and enjoy yourself. Exercise also gives us a purpose. Even when I am having an unproductive day, it is a relief to know that I have done something productive by spending an hour exercising. I have also done something for *myself*, which makes me feel good. If your self-esteem is wavering, exercise is the quickest, most efficient and best way to help.

There can be no better pairing for a healthy life than exercising and eating well. It's better than Posh and Becks, Bogart and Bergman, or Adam and Eve. If you don't begin and get with the programme, you will be in the queue for some of life's other famous pairings: idleness and obesity; osteoporosis and heart disease; and illness and depression.

I received the following email from a friend and it made me laugh out loud. There is nothing like gallows humour to encourage you to face up to the truth that you will need to incorporate regular exercise into your lifestyle if you want to avoid being the woman hunched over in pain, tottering to the corner shop to pick up a pint of milk.

Subject: IMPORTANT MESSAGE

More women need to be aware of this problem …

You've heard about people who have been abducted and had their kidneys removed by black-market organ thieves.

My thighs were stolen from me during the night a few years ago. I went to sleep and woke up with someone else's thighs. It was just that quick. The replacements had the texture of cooked oatmeal. Whose thighs were these and what happened to mine? I spent the entire summer looking for my thighs.

Finally, hurt and angry, I resigned myself to living out my life in jeans. And then the thieves struck again. My butt was next. I knew it was the same gang because they took pains to match my new rear end to the thighs they had stuck me with earlier.

But my new butt was attached at least three inches lower than my original! I realised I'd have to give up my jeans in favour of long skirts.

Two years ago I realised my arms had been switched. One morning I was fixing my hair and was horrified to see the flesh of my upper arm swing to and fro with the motion of the hair-brush. This was really getting scary – my body was being replaced one section at a time. What could they do to me next?

When my poor neck suddenly disappeared and was replaced with a turkey neck, I decided to tell my story.

Women of the world, wake up and smell the coffee! Those plastic surgeons are using real replacement body parts – stolen from you and me! The next time someone you know has something 'lifted', look again – was it lifted from you?

PS: Last year I thought someone had stolen my boobs. I was lying in bed and they were gone! But when I jumped out of bed I was relieved to see that they had just been hiding in my armpits as I slept. Now I keep them hidden in my waistband.

If your brain works like mine, I think the best approach is to tell you why this isn't negotiable. If you exercise six times a week, your body you will grow stronger, more flexible and healthier. When you decide to give yourself the gift of exercising six days a week, you will be helping yourself to stave off obesity, osteoporosis, arthritis, diabetes, heart disease, heart attacks and depression. You can either look and act like a healthy older person who is embracing life's challenges, or you can act and sound like someone who is waiting to grow old. The choice is yours.

Why exercise almost every day of the week?

Exercise increases your circulation and delivers freshly oxygenated blood to all parts of your body – including tissues that may be suffering from lack of oestrogen, such as your skin. Every year more post-menopausal women die of heart disease than all cancers combined. After the age of 65, as many women die of heart attacks as men. I still haven't convinced you and you want more reasons to exercise?

Exercise also ...

- Changes the shape of your body, so your clothes will look better and you will like looking at yourself. This is one step towards reducing feelings of depression and other moments of self-loathing.

- Boosts your metabolism (and keeps it at a higher level for hours after exercising), but it creates muscle that burns fat.

- Encourages restful sleep.

- Improves muscle tone and sore joints that may be causing you pain or discomfort. When it hurts to move, it is close to impossible to enjoy life.

- Improves your sex drive. If you feel better about your body, you are going to want to share it with your partner.

- Keeps you feeling physically and mentally young. Regular exercise improves brain function, including memory, and enhances your emotional well-being by relieving mood swings and helping to relieve the symptoms of depression. Exercise is a natural anti-depressant because it increases serotonin levels, and also encourages the release of feel-good chemicals known as endorphins.

- Reduces your risk of degenerative illnesses associated with ageing, including heart disease, stroke, diabetes and osteoporosis.

- Naturally lowers your blood pressure and cholesterol levels.

- Lowers the risk of some cancers, including breast and colon cancer.

- Improves skin tone and maintains skin elasticity by increasing blood flow to it. Exercise also encourages sweating, which triggers the production of sebum, the skin's own natural moisturiser.

> ❢ Yesterday is history, tomorrow is a mystery, today is God's gift. That is why it is called the present. ❣ *Joan Rivers, entertainer*

Getting started

There are three components to any 30-minute workout:

1. WARMING UP

Every single exercise session should be preceded by a warm-up. If you rush into exercise without warming up your muscles, you're going to hurt yourself. You need 5–10 minutes to get your blood flowing, loosen up your joints, get your spine mobile and aligned, and your brain in the right place for exercise. Try to stretch every part of your body from your neck down to your feet, and push yourself. It's also helpful to involve some more dynamic activity – doing swimming strokes with your arms, or trying out a little skipping or jumping jacks. The idea is simply to get your body going so that you can progress seamlessly into your next activity. The time you allocate to warming up will depend on the time you have allocated to exercise (hence the range of 5–10 minutes).

2. AEROBIC OR STRENGTH TRAINING

Make time to give yourself a full 20-minutes of either aerobic or strength training.

Aerobic or cardiovascular exercise is the key to burning fat and ensuring a healthy pumping heart. Exercise such as brisk walking, swimming, tennis, cross-country skiing, football, swimming, running, cycling, canoeing, kayaking, rowing, back-packing, hiking, low-impact aerobics (the sort you might do in a class), cross-training, spinning and dancing (anything from ballroom, jazz and zumba to barefoot boogie) will all help to increase your heart rate.

Strength or resistance training gives you strong muscles, which will give you a healthier heart, greater endurance levels and lower blood pressure. Strong muscles protect your joints and your back; more muscle power means you put less strain on joints and connective tissue when lifting or exerting your-self. This is important both for treating and preventing arthritis and the general wear and tear associated with ageing. Pilates, yoga, Gyrotonics, TRX suspension training, the phys-ioball, hand-weights and bands all help to integrate strength and improve coordination, while building muscle tone, stamina and a strong and healthy body (more on all of this a little later).

3. COOLING DOWN

Stretch for 5–10 minutes. Regular, careful stretching prevents injury and eases stiff sore muscles.

Aerobic training

My body was designed for a lot of things, but I was simply not made for running. My husband and two daughters had to hold back their giggles when they watched me attempt to jog. You can imagine my joy when I discovered the elliptical cross-trainer.

For the first time in my life I could run 6–8 kilometres without having to worry about knee problems or aching joints. It is an aerobic exercise that works for me.

You will have to find what works for you. You might like the idea of a gym, which can be very sociable. Once you have joined, sign up for as many classes as you can, swim some laps and try out all the machines on offer. Actually joining a gym is a great first step, but you have to remember to go and to use its facilities regularly. Ask for a tour and see if you think it is a place you will enjoy going to most days. Many gyms offer a free trial membership, so take advantage of ongoing promotional offers.

Perhaps you would prefer to put on a pair of trainers and meet a friend to walk your dog in the park. This is a great choice if you are similar to most women in the world and need to multi-task. If you are sweating and feel breathless, but still able to talk, you've hit the right pace. Alternatively, if having a clean home is what makes you happiest, hoover energetically and tackle the dirt with gusto!

There are literally hundreds of ways to get your heart rate up. Some are more fun than others (you just have to use your imagination) and some may be more appropriate to your fitness level. The more you move your body, the quicker your body responds. You will begin to look forward to your exercise sessions – to the point where you crave them. You will start to feel better, and, yes, your butt will become smaller, your clothes will fit better, you will have improved your overall health and fitness and given yourself the opportunity to transform the next 40 years of your life.

YOUR TARGET HEART RATE

To make the most of your aerobic exercise sessions, you need to maintain your heart rate at the correct intensity for you for at least 20 minutes. If your heart rate is too high, your activity can be counterproductive; too low, and you won't experience the aerobic benefits. It takes five minutes to get your heart rate up to your target and then about five minutes for it to return to resting levels, so each session will take about 30 minutes from beginning to end.

If you can invest in a heart-rate monitor (it looks like a watch that you attach to your wrist, and a small stretch belt that you place under your breasts), it will help you to establish if you are exercising at the right intensity without having to stop and take your pulse. If you can't afford to buy one, simply take your pulse by pressing the tips of your index and middle fingers against the inside of the opposite wrist, just below the mound at the base of your thumb. Count how many pulses you feel in a 15-second period. Multiply this number by four to get your heart rate.

Age	Target heart rate (beats per minute)
40	126–153
50	119–145
60	112–136
70	105–128
80	98–119

START SLOWLY

If you are fairly inactive, overweight, or really have not done much exercise in the past five years, do not begin with a high-impact step or kick-boxing class or a 10-kilometre run. Be clever. Start slowly and gradually increase the duration and intensity of your aerobic sessions. Walk instead of drive. The best advice is to push yourself a little – walking a little faster or a little longer every day until you reach your target heart rate for 20 minutes. Walk home and carry your own shopping bags. Take the stairs instead of the lift. See how long you can stand on one foot. Give your children or grandchildren a piggy-back in the park.

Maybe you've always dreamt of going out onto the dance floor and wowing everyone with a fantastic routine. Do it! Enrol yourself in a class, fulfil a fantasy and start getting fit. If you enjoy cycling, jump on your bike and ride everywhere you can. If the great outdoors is your thing, join a hiking or rambling club or take up cross-country skiing or tennis. Whatever you choose, you need to get out there, expand your horizons and feel a sense of accomplishment.

Finding something you actually enjoy will make it that much easier to keep at it for the rest of your life. Mix and match the activities that are the most fun for you. Find a teacher or a trainer you really connect with. Remember, you are only human. Putting in place an exercise routine that you enjoy will ensure that even if you temporarily fall off the wagon, you'll jump back on and begin again.

Forget the ultimate fat-burning routine – it does not exist. If you don't enjoy it, you will do it two or three times and never do it again. Making exercise a regular part of your daily routine will make the biggest difference in how you grow older. Exercise can and will change your life.

When you start to enjoy your aerobic sessions and find that you are getting fitter by the day, you can then think about increasing the length and frequency of your sessions. Make sure you treat yourself to some nice workout clothes and a gym bag. Good workout clothes immediately make you look half a stone lighter and can give you the motivation to get started.

THE THRILL OF COMPETITION

Competitive sports will rekindle a dormant killer instinct while improving your overall physical and mental health. Competition encourages us to learn how to handle conflict, strive for success, recognise and accept failure, and communicate. In some ways, it mirrors life. So many of us gave up competitive sports back in our teens and early 20s. I think you will be surprised how playing to win improves your mind, spirit and body. Lose your worries in the thrill of competition.

FEEL AND LOOK PHYSICALLY YOUNGER

Aerobic exercise should make you feel good on many levels. As well as giving you more physical strength and balance, it can help you to express your emotions, provide you with an opportunity to socialise and meet people, improve your balance, let your body communicate through music and movement, help sharpen your mind by having to remember a step or dance routine, and give you a chance to have a good laugh – either at yourself or with others. You will feel like you have cleaned out years of mental cobwebs, making you a happier person who looks and feels physically younger too!

Strength and resistance training

Sometimes it is important to state the obvious. Even if you are the most unfit person in the world – and by that I mean you haven't properly exercised for a few years or you have put on so much weight that you are buying and wearing clothes that are several sizes bigger than you used to – you *do not* qualify for a 'get out of jail' card when it comes to strength training. There are absolutely no excuses not to begin.

If there is a voice in your head that is already saying, 'I can't possibly exercise six times a week,' silence it! Make some changes to the way you organise your time. Do your weekly shop on the internet and get your groceries delivered, wake up half an hour earlier in the morning, close your office door and take some time to work out during your lunch break. It's all about priorities. If you can find 30 minutes to watch your favourite soap, you can find the same for exercise. In fact, you can strength-train *and* watch *Coronation Street* or your favourite repeats of *Dr Who* at the same time.

Looking in the mirror and liking what you see is important too. Strength training will give you strong muscles that will improve the way you look. Lean muscles are taut against your body, as opposed to flab, which hangs off the bone and makes you look a lot fatter than you actually are. Resistance training will help to burn fat and calories. The good news is this allows you to eat a little more (not junk food) and retain your healthy weight. It also means that the food you do eat is burnt off rather than being laid down as fat. Your metabolism will improve too. Muscle tissue burns as much as 15 times more calories per day than fat, even when you are sleeping and reading the newspaper! It's not about weight you see on the scales. You may only lose a couple of kilos, but you will change the shape of your body and lose inches all over. It's not unusual to drop two dress sizes within a couple of months of training.

Feel and see the benefits

When it comes to the health of your heart, mental agility and fat-burning, aerobic exercise is the way to go. When it comes to body stability, posture, flexibility, healthy joints, bone density and improving the way that you look, strength training is your soul sister.

With a bit of luck, your life will be not only long but ageless and painless. You want to stay healthy, active and very mobile. By looking after yourself and exercising six times a week, the inner you will start to feel years younger.

Visualise how you want to act, look and feel 25 or 40 years from now. Exercise is not just necessary but essential until the day you die. Build a solid aerobic base, muscle strength and healthy joints one day at a time for the rest of your life.

Find the best routine for you

So what's the best type of strength training for you? I surveyed over 200 women about the type of exercise they enjoy most, and Pilates came in a strong first, followed by yoga, Gyrotonics®, the power plate, t'ai chi, Bosu® balance trainer, ABS on the physioball, TRX® suspension and finally weight training. If this all sounds like something in a foreign language, read on! All these forms of strength training are widely available. The internet will be able to help you find classes nearest to where you live.

About two years ago, I decided to try Pilates. After years of step classes, working out in the gym, playing tennis, swimming and sharing a personal trainer twice a week, I finally found the exercise that works best for me and my body: dynamic Pilates.

Dynamic Pilates

Imagine all the legendary silhouette-sleeking power of Pilates, but with the cardiovascular benefits of an aerobics class or a step workout. Also imagine feeling amazing and seeing results in just 10 sessions. According to David Higgins, co-founder of Ten Pilates, 'Like traditional Pilates, dynamic Pilates is designed to strengthen and engage your core waist and lower back muscles, buttocks and diaphragm, helping to improve posture and prevent injury. Unlike traditional Pilates, dynamic Pilates delivers an innovative, intense and highly effective full-body workout designed to give you a slimmer figure and lean, toned muscles. And it works quickly. After about five sessions you really can start to see a difference. After 10 sessions, your husband and girlfriends will see a difference too.'

Joseph Pilate, the creator of Pilates, had a strong belief in the mind–body relationship and understood that a fit, healthy body is the key to an agile, healthy mind. He said, 'You will feel better in 10 sessions, look better in 20 sessions and have a completely new body in 30 sessions.' With dynamic Pilates you can achieve all this in half the time!

Pilates is the best, most efficient workout for tightening up your bottom and stomach, toning your thighs, calves and arms, and giving your muscles definition you could previously only dream of having. Plus, it helps with injury prevention, relieves chronic backache, straightens your spine, improves your posture and keeps your muscles flexible. My husband now takes part too. It was difficult to convince him to attend a class the first time (we told him Claudia Schiffer would be there), but once he was there, he quickly found muscles he didn't know he had and that his über personal trainer was actually a wimp compared to his new Pilates instructor.

Stars and celebrities have been touting the virtues of Pilates for years. Kate Winslet attributes her svelte and toned body to doing 30-minute sessions of Pilates three or four times a week. Everyone from Jennifer Aniston to Dame Joan Bakewell swears by it. Start by finding a Pilates studio where they teach dynamic Pilates and watch your body shape change in six weeks at the most.

Yoga

Yoga is designed to connect the mind, body and spirit, and there are several different types. For example, Iyengar is slow and precise, while Ashtanga (sometimes referred to as 'power yoga') is quicker and more fluid. It works the entire body equally, including your legs, stomach, arms, back and core muscles. Meditation and chanting is included for free!

Yoga's popularity has soared because, once connected with its magic, we feel supple and 'open'. Most of us want to move and feel like we did when we were younger, and for women over the age of 50, this is one of the ways to achieve it.

Faced with physical injury, stiff joints and limbs, yoga 'greases' your engine! As the mind focuses on posture, your body will let go into the movement. Once you find your way, the mind and body usually begin to crave more of the practice. Like all commitments, there is a discipline and patience involved. The yoga experience must be viewed as an ongoing part of your life.

Gyrotonics®

Friends in Los Angeles claim that the Gyrotonic method has now overtaken Pilates as one of the most popular forms of exercise. Watch this space – it is going to get even bigger here. Gyrotonic exercises employ movements from swimming, yoga, Pilates, gymnastics and t'ai chi, using specialised equipment developed by Juliu Horvath, the creator of Gyrotonics. The system is intended to improve flexibility and balance, as well as muscle strength, and to increase overall stability and mobility in the joints. It offers three-dimensional, circular movements that use yogic breathing patterns to clean, detoxify and rejuvenate the entire body.

The Gyrotonic tower machines simultaneously stretch and strengthen muscles and tendons, while also mobilising the joints. Corresponding breathing patterns are used during the exercises, increasing coordination, endurance and aerobic activity. The exercises are complementary to Pilates and there are several studios that specialise in this method of strength training.

Power plate

Exercising on a power plate is very effective for increasing strength, stability and flexibility, as well as improving your circulation and range of motion. When done vigorously, it's great cardiovascular (aerobic) exercise. It involves using a machine that vibrates to enhance your workout. It can be used at various speeds, which also makes it effective in physical rehabilitation after an accident, surgery or stroke, for example.

The technology it uses was invented by NASA to enable astronauts to remain fit in space, despite being in very confined quarters with little gravity. The basic principle is that you do typical exercise moves (such as lunges, squats, push-ups, plank, tricep dips and crunches), but on a platform that is vibrating 30–60 times per second. The instability caused by the rapid vibration requires your core muscles to do more with each move, and calls on a wider muscle group to 'pitch in'. So each move is far more demanding than it would be on solid ground, which means you get a great workout in half the time.

One other added benefit (perhaps it should have been mentioned first) is that the power plate can cause spontaneous orgasms, thanks to the wonderful vibration that it transmits through the entire body. Now that's reason enough to sign up for a few classes!

T'ai chi

A cross between yoga and meditation, t'ai chi consists of a series of graceful movements and breathing exercises designed to build strength, restore balance and increase flexibility, while helping you to attain a heightened state of being. In fact, t'ai chi is more than exercise. If practised correctly and regularly, you can use this ancient exercise as effective alternative healing for a wide range of health problems. The movements involved are designed to circulate your body's invisible energy or 'chi'. Smooth circulation of chi ensures a healthy body and mind, while stagnant or blocked chi is believed to be at the root of all sorts of chronic health problems. Even better, t'ai chi can help to reduce pain and increase mobility in ageing joints, including those affected by arthritis. T'ai chi is often described as 'meditation with movement'.

Bosu® balance trainer

A Bosu is a rubbery, flat-bottomed dome approximately 65 cm wide: it looks like an exercise ball cut in half. Exercising on an uneven surface improves your balance and forces you to use and strengthen deep-core and stabilising muscles. Simply standing on it makes the muscles in your body come alive. Bosu can be integrated into any strength-training routine.

ABS on a physioball

Abdominal, back and stability (ABS) exercises on a physioball are a very efficient way to exercise because devotees believe a healthy back and strong core can be achieved in as little as 20 minutes three times a week. The exercises involve sitting on a large physioball, with your hips and knees at a 90-degree angle. A basic workout includes crunches, plank, knee tucks, balancing on your knees and back extensions. One of the many wonderful things about the physioball is that you can use it at home and it is almost impossible to be in the wrong position. A wrong position means falling off the ball!

TRX® suspension

I love this because it works, but it is *hard*. Developed by the United States Navy Seals (some of the world's finest commandos), the TRX suspension trainer (a pair of stretchy straps that can be anchored to a door, a tree – in fact, anywhere) began as an invention of necessity. On ships and inside submarines, the Seals searched for ways to stay in peak condition while confined to small spaces. Although TRX was originally designed to build strength and muscle wherever you are, you should start your training with an instructor – either one-on-one or in a class. After you get the hang of it, you can buy your own equipment and train at home.

Weight training

Weight training is probably the easiest and cheapest way to strengthen your muscles and achieve overall fitness. It's a good idea to get some help from a trainer at your local gym before embarking on a programme that involves using weights or resistance bands. You will need to learn how to protect your back and how to control your movements to make this workout most effective.

> Always protect your back when doing any form of strength training. You'll need to keep a 'neutral spine', which involves sucking in your tummy and making sure your hips and bottom are tucked in.

There are five exercises that can easily be done in your own home, garden or office (with the door shut!) without any equipment except your own body. These include squats, push-ups, lunges, plank and abdominal crunches. If you are not sure how to do these, http://exercise.about.com will teach you how. Once you become stronger, you can use weights and resistance bands to fatigue your muscles quickly and efficiently. Ultimately, weight training will help you to use your body more easily and effectively.

Start by doing each of these exercises for one minute and then work up to three minutes for each exercise. With five minutes of warm-up and another five minutes of cooling down (stretching), you'll be exercising for just 30 minutes – about the same length of time it takes to colour the roots of your hair.

You will need to purchase a pair of light to medium-weight dumb-bells (about 2.5 kg each). The weights should be light enough to be lifted, but heavy enough to make you need to stop after 8–12 repetitions. Alternatively, you can purchase resistance stretch bands, such as Dyna-Bands®. The general idea is that you secure the band around a fixed point and use it to resist your movement, thereby making it harder and exercising your muscles. Resistance bands can be used for a full-body workout or for exercising each of the main muscle groups.

Remember, walk before you run and build your strength gradually.

Stretch smart

Stretching, or cooling down, is essential after all your exercise sessions. Take 5–10 minutes to do this in order to prevent injury, relieve stiffness and soreness and encourage increased flexibility and range of motion. Hold each stretch for 10–30 seconds, to the point of very minor discomfort. Try not to force any stretch and make sure you stretch your whole body one muscle group at a time: your calves, hamstrings, lower back, chest, shoulders, triceps and neck. Listen to your body; you'll soon know when the stretch has worked.

The bargain of a lifetime

We all know that how we feel dictates our state of mind and vice versa. By choosing to exercise 30 minutes a day, six days a week, you are giving yourself the best chance to live the life you want to live.

A body that is fully functioning will keep you feeling positive, emotionally connected and happy. With that comes a feeling of youth, energy, verve and enthusiasm. A body that is active and engaged every day of the week will give you the strength, optimism and flexibility to do whatever you want and need to do each day.

For all of you out there who think you are too busy to embark on making the rest of your life fun, fulfilling and pain-free, remember this: exercise is a two-for-one deal. By giving yourself a strong and healthy body, you are *choosing* how you want to age and making a serious commitment to your future. Regular exercise lays the foundation for the life you want to live. A body that retires early from living is a wasted one. When you make daily exercise part of your life, you hold one of the keys to a life worth living.

My top 10 tips to change your life

1. Connect with your body by doing something that involves building strength or getting your heart pumping six times a week.

2. Stretch and warm up your muscles before *any* form of exercise.

3. Hire a personal trainer, if it is within your means, even if it is only for one session. It will be a great investment. You will be taught how to exercise and given an idea of the exercises that are right for you. An individually tailored programme can help to keep you motivated.

4. Join a gym, use their machines, take their classes and have one of their trainers assess you and formulate a programme for you. Experiment until you find a class, an exercise routine, a gym or a trainer you really like and then stick with it. If money is short, go for a free trial session to get some ideas for incorporating exercise into your daily life.

5. Find a local class that offers some of the strength-training disciplines discussed on pages 72–6. Classes are motivating and produce clear results. They are also a great opportunity to socialise and well worth the investment. For the price of an inexpensive bottle of wine, which will only make your hot flushes worse and expand your waistline, you can buy yourself a class that could change your life forever.

6. Think back to some of your favourite activities you enjoyed in your youth. Did you surf, cycle, ski, play golf or tennis, or ride a horse? Why not bring them back into your life?

Something you enjoy doing will encourage you to make time for it. If you've never had a passion for sports or exercise, there is no time like today to find one!

7. There are lots of things you can do at home while watching your favourite programmes on television, such as lunges, leg lifts, crunches, tricep dips, weight-lifting and the plank. The most important thing to remember is that these types of exercise are most effective when done regularly. You should push yourself as hard as you can, but *always* protect your back (see page 73).

8. It doesn't cost much to get started. Two dumb-bells, a resistance band and an exercise ball will help you with balance, stability and strength and will keep you going for decades.

9. Remember to breathe. Exhale as you exert yourself and then inhale. Many people hold their breath as they lift or exert themselves, but your cells need oxygen when you exercise. Breathing and breath awareness reduces muscular tension, improves circulation and reduces stress.

10. Make exercise addictive. The more you exercise and the stronger you get, the more your body needs and wants it.

Regular exercise will give you the energy to pursue your new passions and the ability to rediscover the best in yourself. By making this small change to your daily routine, you will be giving yourself the promise of a strong body, the energy to face the world, the chance to make new connections and friendships and the ability to live your life without pain – to help you make the second half of your life the best half.

CHAPTER FOUR

Diet
The noun, not the verb

'This is what learning is. You suddenly understand something you've understood all your life, but in a new way.'

Doris Lessing, author

At this time in your life, you are probably completely preoccupied with the fact you are putting on weight and wondering why you don't own more clothes in your wardrobe with expandable waistbands. For over 95 per cent of women in their peri- or post-menopausal years, gaining weight goes hand-in-hand with losing your hormones.

Why? Quite simply, normal levels of progesterone and oestrogen regulate metabolism, weight gain and water retention, while testosterone regulates appetite and helps the body to create muscle. Our hormones have a direct impact not only on our appetite and metabolism, but also how and where we store fat. That wonderful hourglass figure you've had your whole life will gradually morph into something resembling the shape of an apple.

Stress hormones and hormone imbalances cause weight gain. Insulin starts eating up all the sugar and carbohydrates, and stores it as fat around your middle and on your breasts. That's why there is a dramatic shift in the body's configuration. A bit of added bloat comes with the territory as well. Ultimately, this will give us inner peace but more to hold on to!

If you keep eating as you did in your 30s, expect to gain a minimum of 1 kg a year throughout your menopausal years (peri-menopause up to menopause itself). Girls, that is anywhere from 5–8 kg. Let me make one thing clear: you will *never* get even close to your ideal weight and shape without a two-pronged attack – eating the right foods and increasing the amount you exercise. Research has shown that people who eat well and are in good shape in their 50s are the ones most likely to age well. Wishing, hoping and praying will only get you unhealthier, fatter and more out of shape. If you want to live a long and active life, start today making the small changes necessary to achieve this.

When we were younger we could stay up all night and not have it show on our faces for the next two days. Now we see all too plainly the consequences of staying out late or a heavy night of drinking. Dieting is a lot like this too. We used to be able to cut back on alcohol, carbs or sugar, add a few sessions at the gym, and the weight would melt off. These old tricks just don't work any more. Losing weight is simply much more difficult, despite eating less. Anyone over the age of 48 who says they don't have to watch what they eat is just plain lying or blessed with a rare metabolic disorder or thyroid condition.

The food you eat will be crucially important to the way you age. A diet that is rich in fresh fruit and vegetables, wholegrains, good-quality proteins and essential fatty acids will not only help to prevent many of the degenerative effects of ageing and some of the symptoms of menopause, but will also give your body the nutrients it needs to operate efficiently. Being overweight is linked to a host of debilitating diseases, including type 2 diabetes, cardiovascular disease, hypertension, high cholesterol, stroke, osteoarthritis, breathing problems, some types of cancer and urinary incontinence.

So when you think 'diet', think of the noun, not the verb. Most women battle for years with their weight, losing it and putting it back on, or finding that they can't lose it at all. I am a self-proclaimed expert on diets. I have tried all of them, from Atkins and Montignac to South Beach, Scarsdale and Cabbage

Soup (to name just a few!). I would lose the weight and gain it right back again.

I have learned that your diet should focus on eating the right food to protect bone health, using the right fats (see page 91), keeping your alcohol consumption in check, drinking enough water to keep you hydrated, and eating unprocessed foods (preferably organic) that are fresh and as close to their natural state as possible.

Dieting does not work

We are old enough, wise enough and have tried enough diets to know that dieting does not work. Scientists have been striving for decades to work out a diet that will not only help us lose weight, but keep weight off. There is a big and growing market (maybe because big and growing is what we are becoming) based around diverse theories on how to become slim. Yet not one person, one institute, one association or even one study can agree on a long-term weight-loss formula that is predictable or consistent.

Even the most tried-and-tested formula – cut down on calories and lose weight – becomes less effective over time because the body just becomes more efficient at conserving energy (calories). Despite all the new technology and inventions of the past 100 years, scientists have not been able to come up with a better way of quantifying the fattening nature of food than the calorie, a unit of energy first measured under crude laboratory conditions over a century ago. The latest research, from nutritionist Geoffrey Livesey, proves that all calories are not created equal. Where is that on the food labelling?

If you have dieted in the past by counting calories, you need to think about the following fact: texture, cooking and fibre content can alter the number of calories your body extracts from food.

Counting calories

Calorie counting was first developed in the late 19th century by an American chemist, Wilbur Olin Atwater. He calculated energy content by burning small samples of food in controlled conditions and measured the amount of energy released in the form of heat. With few modifications, these measurements have been the currency of food ever since. Using just a little bit of common sense should lead you to the conclusion that calorie counting is an obsolete and absurd approach to losing weight – we all know our bodies don't incinerate food, but digest it!

I think most consumers are confused by food labelling. Don't fool yourself into thinking that all food is created equal – 250 calories of fresh fruit is *not* the same as 250 calories of chocolate. Remember, Mr Atwater's test tubes did not take into account texture, fibre or how food has been processed and cooked. The body burns raw foods faster than cooked food, so the calories in your melon, your salad or your crudités will be burned off long before those contained in a chocolate brownie or a bowl of ice cream. Also, the nutrients contained in the raw foods far exceed those in the processed ones.

You may need to set new goals when it comes to your diet. Simply said, your diet should consist primarily of unprocessed foods because you will burn them faster, they are less likely to be laid down as fat, and they will provide you with many of the nutrients you need for optimum health and well-being.

An epidemic of fat

So why has obesity become a generational phenomenon that started around the mid-1980s? When I grew up, there were maybe one or two fat kids out of the hundreds of children in the school playground. Our mothers didn't spend their time spinning at the gym, taking Pilates classes and power-walking around the park, but they were slim, with lovely cinched waists, and could pretty much eat what and when they wanted.

By the mid-1960s, Wimpy bars and Kentucky Fried Chicken outlets appeared alongside traditional fish and chip shops across the UK, and in 1974 McDonalds arrived. There was also plenty of chocolate on offer: Flakes, Buttons, Kit-Kats, Smarties, Maltesers, Milk Tray, Mars Bars and more. Ready-made meals began to appear, and started the gradual decline in home cooking. Bottled water did not exist.

Are we getting fatter because food is readily available and cheap? Or could it be what is happening to our food before it gets into our mouths?

State-of-the-art exercise equipment, such as the cross-trainer, rowing machine, treadmill and power plate, did not exist. People wore plimsolls, while nowadays there are bespoke hi-tech shoes for each and every exercise known to mankind. Personal trainers were for Olympic athletes, not for your average man and woman just looking to get fit. So what has changed? It wasn't as if we were super-healthy back in the 1950s and 1960s, but we certainly weren't fat. Today even the healthiest and fittest people struggle with their weight.

If in the 'good old days' we could eat whatever and whenever we wanted and not gain weight, could it be that the change we are seeing has its roots in the way that our food is produced? Houses and cars cost 14 times what they did 50 years ago, but the price of chicken hasn't even doubled. Does it make you pause and wonder why you can buy a whole chicken at the supermarket for less than it costs to get a latte at Starbucks?

Getting food-smart

You will never see an advertisement on television promoting the nutritional wonders of a fresh apple or a bunch of celery. But manufacturers can make sugar-frosted cornflakes or chocolate pops sound like the most nutritious option of the day. In England we spend more than £300 million a year on cereal bars, believing they are good for us. In fact, the average bar has more than eight teaspoons of sugar per 100 g. Hopefully, you are too smart for this, but if you've been conned in the past, it's worth bearing this in mind: fresh foods that are unprocessed and unrefined should be the mainstay of your diet.

According to Megan Patel, a leader in the field of natural health and founder of the Hank Society, an organic food company, 'By feeding your body unrefined, easily digestible, nutrient-rich food, you will never ever have to calorie count or be afraid that what you put in your mouth will end up around your middle. When you properly feed your body you feel much more satisfied and, here is the bonus, you eat less.'

Much of the food we eat has been grown and reared in a different way than it was when we were growing up. This has had an impact on our overall health – and our waistlines. Due to the rise of factory farming and the use of additives and chemicals, food has become much cheaper in real terms. This means that our weekly food shop today is a smaller percentage of the average family's budget than it was in 1960. Fifty years ago, food did not have anything like the amount of preservatives it does today. Our mothers shopped daily at their local butcher and greengrocer, and kept little food in the house. Children were told they needed to eat more to grow big and strong. Now 'big' is a national epidemic.

Although supermarkets boast good-quality products at rock-bottom prices, have you ever looked at the list of ingredients that go into, for example, a Victoria sponge cake? The ingredients are largely unrecognisable in any language.

Governments spend enormous amounts of our tax pounds reassuring us that farmers employ safe practices; however, the goalposts have shifted. What is now considered to be safe is very different from what it was even 50 years ago. We have genetically modified foods, animals routinely fed antibiotics, and even beef full of growth-enhancers if it's shipped in from America. A bewildering number of chemicals in the form of colourings, preservatives, appearance enhancers and more are added to our food to keep it looking better for longer.

In Jonathan Safran Foer's book *Eating Animals*, he explores farming practices in the USA, and how the raising and killing of birds and farm animals have created many of the health problems we live with today. He writes:

‘Why are entire flocks of industrial, intensively reared birds dying at once? And what about the people eating those birds? Just the other day, a local paediatrician was telling me he's seeing all kinds of illnesses that he never used to see. Not only juvenile diabetes, but inflammatory and auto-immune diseases that a lot of the doctors don't even know what to call. And girls are going through puberty much earlier, and kids are allergic to just about everything, and asthma is out of control. Everyone knows it's our food. We're messing with the genes of these animals and feeding them growth hormones and all kinds of drugs that we really don't know enough about. Then we're eating them. Kids today are the first generation to grow up on this stuff, and we're making a science experiment out of them.’

To summarise, I think your new diet should consist of the very best-quality food you can afford, organic if possible, grown on farms in your local area or bought from your local farmers' market. Buy meat from butchers known to have good food practices. If you have the time, try to buy your produce daily to preserve its nutrients. (Food in the supermarket has usually spent a while in the back of a lorry or in a warehouse somewhere, thus compromising its nutritional value.) Eating foods in their most natural state will help you to maximise the benefits of the food you are putting in your body. This, combined with exercise, should help you to lose weight, feel better and enjoy looking at the person staring back at you in the mirror.

Organic apple cider vinegar

Haven't you always wanted to know how to lose the first 2kg and keep it off without starving yourself, taking laxatives, sitting in a steam room for a few hours a day or having a colonic? Here's a way of losing the first kilo or two without any hardship that I hope will put you on the road to making other changes in your day-to-day life. It's completely natural, it's organic and it's sold at health-food shops everywhere. Do I have your attention? It's apple cider vinegar (ACV), and what it does is put your body into a slightly alkaline state that encourages healthy cell function and helps combat fatigue and disease. According to Dr Susan E Brown and Larry Trivieri, Jr in *The Acid–Alkaline Food Guide,* 'When the body is in a lightly alkaline state, it allows for an easy flow of oxygen and nutrients into the cell walls and an equally easy disposal of cellular waste.'

I had been trying to lose the same 4kg for the past seven years. The vicious cycle of losing the weight and putting it back on was getting more difficult, so I decided to 'be sensible'. I hired a personal trainer twice a week. I played tennis at least once a week. I cut back on the amount of carbohydrates I ate. I cut back on the amount of meat I ate. I drastically cut back on the amount of sugar that went into my body. But every time I got on the scales, my weight was basically the same – or creeping up a kilo or so in the wrong direction.

Then I met an incredibly glamorous and fit 54-year-old on holiday and I asked her to tell me her secret. She said that she exercised six times a week. 'Isn't that too much?' I asked. 'My trainer said two to three times.' She smiled and repeated herself: 'Six times a week.'

So I upped the number of exercise sessions to five and then six days a week. I enrolled in four Pilates classes (dynamic Pilates, the hard kind I wrote about in Chapter 3, which combines aerobic and strength training), and managed two additional aerobic sessions a week. My body definitely started to change shape. Friends would ask me if I had lost weight, but when I weighed myself, I could not even boast that I had lost a single gram.

I started to believe that I would have to resign myself to the fact that weight gain is just part of getting older, learn to accept it and be happy with what was good in my life. There was plenty to be happy about. The shape and size of my body was as good as it was ever going to get. I really needed to start focusing my energy on something that I might actually be able to change about myself.

I was having a small moan about all of this to a gorgeous, incredibly stylish and thin Chinese friend and *eureka*! She said that she was a big believer in organic apple cider vinegar (ACV), which is used to speed up metabolism and suppress appetite naturally. She had been using it for years and thought it was a great natural cleanser, too.

I decided to look into it, and discovered that Hippocrates, the 'father of medicine', used it for its health benefits as long ago as 400 BC. Julius Caesar's army used it to stay healthy and fight off disease. Samurai warriors drank it for strength. And – surprise, surprise – it has been used as a weight-loss remedy for centuries. I began using it and within two weeks I had lost a little over 1 kg – weight that I had been trying to lose for the past four years. By the end of a month I had lost 2.5 kg. I was ecstatic.

The ACV that I want you to buy is unfiltered and unpasteurised, and contains no preservatives. Because it is made from raw organic apples, there are no health risks. Diet pills make you jumpy and shaky, can change your personality and are bad for your health. Organic ACV is actually more effective than diet pills because it not only reduces appetite, but also breaks down fat and gets the entire metabolism going. My friends have also been converted and cannot believe how quickly it works.

I don't know why it works and shifts pounds off your body weight, but I can tell you that ACV:

- Makes the body burn calories more efficiently.

- Reduces cravings and overall appetite.

- Gets the entire metabolism working again.

- Will result in weight loss of about 2kg in just one month.

Start with just one teaspoon of ACV mixed with 300ml hot or warm water in the morning and early evening (around 5 p.m.). If you don't like the taste, mix about 50ml apple juice into your water, or stir your ACV into a smoothie. After about four weeks, once your body has adjusted, you can increase the amount of ACV to two teaspoons morning and evening. Do *not* be tempted to think more is better. It is not, and can make you feel extremely nauseous.

The health benefits of ACV are extensive. In addition to weight loss, it has been claimed that ACV is effective in curing menopausal symptoms such as night sweats and hot flushes, as well as other female conditions such as Candida and urinary tract infections. It is also credited with curing allergies, arthritis, asthma, cholesterol, colds, coughs, diabetes, eczema, headaches, heartburn, leg cramps, and can lower high blood pressure. I don't know about all of this; what I do know is that it is an easy way to jump-start your new, healthy diet.

Eat well, be well

Menopause is hard enough without making your life a complete misery. It would be cruel to suggest that you could never again have a lovely piece of triple-chocolate cake or treacle pudding. However, you need to be realistic – and 'realistic' is the operative word. If you eat well, exercise regularly in the right way for your body, and change your eating habits just a little, you can eat a bowl of ice cream (or even two) and not gain an ounce or compromise your health.

If you think eating a fry-up followed by sticky toffee pudding and a cappuccino sprinkled with chocolate can ever be more than a *very* occasional treat, stop, and put this book down now. Waddle to the mirror and check out your very large backside and jelly belly. Then say to yourself, 'I will make some minor adjustments so I can live a long, healthy and happy life and not look, act or be old before my time.'

Make vegetables your mainstay

Research has shown that populations eating a plant-based diet are far less likely to be overweight or obese. They also experience lower rates of heart disease, diabetes, high blood pressure and other life-threatening diseases. According to a recent study of more than 55,000 Swedish women by Tufts University researcher P. Kirstin Newby, 40 per cent of meat-eaters were overweight compared to only 25–29 per cent of vegetarians and vegans.

I am not trying to turn you into a vegan. I am simply asking you to put a lot more vegetables on your plate and a lot less chicken, lamb and beef – and even certain fish (see below). Protein is important and your body needs it for muscle development, to build and repair tissues, and to make enzymes, hormones and other body chemicals. It's also necessary for bones, cartilage, skin and blood. However, you don't need to get all your protein from animal products. Plant-based proteins, such as chickpeas, lentils, beans and other pulses, as well as the grain quinoa, mean you can mix and match your proteins. A small fist-sized portion of protein at breakfast, lunch and dinner is all you need. Because fish is so rich in healthy essential fatty acids, it is an ideal form of protein. This is part of the problem. Our love affair with seafood and the profound effects of overfishing has brought about an imminent extinction of the bluefish tuna and other fish, such as cod. If you haven't seen the movie *End of the Line*, you must. It's the reason for my reticence in recommending a lot of fish in your diet.

How big is your plate and what's on it?

Fill half your plate with salad and/or vegetables, and then devote a quarter each to other healthy protein and whole-grain carbohydrates. Not only will this help to ensure a balance of nutrients, but it will put the focus firmly on vegetables to balance your weight.

Think about the size of your plate, too. Instead of serving meals on a dinner plate, think about using a side plate. This means you are not tempted to 'supersize' your portions. The healthiest 80-year-old couple I know have been doing this for 20 years.

Keep a food diary

Most people have no idea what they put in their mouths every day. You might be surprised at the number of calories you inadvertently put in yours. A few women I spoke with who have kept weight off for more than a year said it was the best way to see where and when they were piling on the weight. Keep a detailed food diary for at least a week. It will probably solve the riddle of your expanding waistline.

ACID AND ALKALINE

When doctors and nutritionists encourage you to 'alkalise your blood', they usually suggest eating plenty of fresh vegetables, which have an alkaline-forming effect on your system. The reason for this is that many years spent eating a poor diet (rich in white-flour products and sugars) creates acid conditions in your blood. Your kidneys, lungs and skin must work overtime to balance the body's pH – in other words, the balance between alkaline and acid. It does this by borrowing alkaline minerals, such as calcium and potassium, from bone and tissue.

Over the long haul, an acidic diet means that bones and muscles are weakened and ageing is accelerated. Osteoporosis, muscle loss, joint issues and back problems are associated with slightly acidic states. In fact, acid conditions will decrease your body's ability to absorb minerals and other nutrients, lower its ability to repair damaged cells, decrease energy production in the cells, encourage the growth of some cancers, and make you more susceptible to fatigue and illness.

A diet rich in vegetables will help to keep your body's alkaline/acid balance at the right level. Most people love vegetables when they are cooked in appealing, appetising and inventive ways. When you were little your mother definitely made you eat your vegetables, so there must be a few that you like.

Many vegetables, particularly the brightly coloured varieties, are high in antioxidants and nutrients. The truth is, however, that all vegetables are good for you, particularly when they are eaten raw, steamed or cooked without any sauces.

Note: Your twice-a-day drink of organic apple cider vinegar will also help you to achieve the correct alkaline balance.

Boost your fibre intake

Fibre is a nutrient. It acts as a broom to clean out your system and encourages healthy digestion. The best sources of fibre are wholegrains, pulses, seeds, fresh fruit and vegetables. I love adding two teaspoons of flaxseeds (high in vitamin B, magnesium, omega-3 fatty acids, fibre and phyto-chemicals) to my low-fat probiotic yoghurt or cottage cheese every morning. Flaxseed is one of the most perfect nutrients on the planet, combining healthy fat and high fibre.

Not all fats are created equal

Depending where it comes from, not all fat is bad. Fats are necessary in your diet, but it is the *type* of fat that matters most. There are basically two types.

Saturated fat is found in animal products and some plant-based foods, such as coconut and palm oil. Trans fats are a subdivision of saturated fats: they start out unsaturated but become saturated when the food industry adds hydrogen to harden them and prolong shelf life. Whatever their origin, saturated fats raise the bad cholesterol (LDL) in your blood, block your arteries and lower your good cholesterol (HDL).

Unsaturated fat is subdivided into monounsaturates (found in olive, rapeseed and peanut oils, and avocados),and polyunsaturates (found in fish, flaxseed, walnuts and plant food, such as corn oil). Both types raise your good (HDL) cholesterol and serve as a Dyno-Rod for your arteries. They also act as natural anti-inflammatories, balancing hormones, maintaining blood-sugar levels and healthy metabolism, lowering bad (LDL) cholesterol, encouraging healthy hair and skin, regulating thyroid activity, boosting immunity and ensuring the healthy functioning of the brain and nervous system. The main difference between mono- and polyunsaturates is that mono-unsaturates do not achieve these benefits so efficiently.

> ## Warning about nuts
>
> Although nuts are definitely a healthy option, filled with mono- and polyunsaturated fats and powerful antioxidants, they should only be eaten in moderation and unsalted. Athletes who are trying to bulk up say that nuts are their preferred snack food, so unless you are capable of eating just a handful and putting the bag away, choose another food to snack on.

White is not a good colour, even in summer

Stay away from all white foods – white flour, white bread, white pasta, white rice and white potatoes. They are nutritional lightweights, short on vitamins, fibre and minerals.

Sugar is the devil

Sugar's destructive ability goes well beyond calories and making you fat. It depresses your immune system, raises your cholesterol, creates an acidic digestive environment, lowers your sex drive and attacks the collagen that is left in your body, thereby prematurely ageing your skin. Look at labels for lurking evils, such as fructose and corn syrup, and try to avoid all of the obvious processed sugars found in pre-packed foods. Although we all know there is zero nutritional value to sugar, there is one primary reason why we eat it. It tastes good. It's a drug for our taste buds. Make a big effort to keep away from it.

Go green

Phytoestrogens are a group of chemicals found in plants that can act like the hormone oestrogen. During menopause, oestrogen starts to decline, which can lead to many of the symptoms of menopause, and also to osteoporosis and high cholesterol. Phytoestrogens are particularly useful for menopausal women and some studies show that they reduce the symptoms of menopause significantly. Soya beans are by far the best source, but other good sources include wholegrains, beans, nuts, seeds, seed oils, berries, fruits, vegetables and roots. One way to introduce them easily into your life is to use soya milk whenever you can – in your scrambled eggs, porridge or even latte. If you don't like the taste, hide it in foods where it isn't noticeable.

Drink water – and make it tap!

Aim to drink 6–8 glasses of water every day. I know it is hard to remember, but if you keep a large jug of water on your bedside table, in your sitting room or on the desk in your office, you might remember to drink it. Water is important for a number of reasons. First and foremost, keeping your body well hydrated will encourage it to function more effectively. You will also experience higher energy levels, better hair and skin, regular bowel movements, optimum kidney function, lubricated joints and stronger immunity. Filtered tap water is over 99 per cent pure and you don't have to pay for it. In this case, one of the best things in life is free.

Coping with cravings

In 1668 the French actor and playwright Molière said it best: 'One must eat to live, not live to eat.' Unless somebody is nominating you for sainthood any time soon, you must indulge your cravings occasionally. It is tough enough being a post-menopausal woman without giving up the odd sinful pleasure.

We are only human. However, if you have a BMI over 27 (see page 51), you are putting yourself in dangerous health territory. Talk to your doctor. You might need help when it comes to losing weight and following the 'exercise more, eat less' mantra.

Anti-obesity drugs have, unfortunately, had mixed results, producing serious side effects in some people. For this reason, I offer no advice here, except to consult your doctor.

Foods that play havoc with your hormones

- **Sugar-free drinks and snacks.** Most food labelled 'sugar-free' contains artificial sweeteners and other additives that create a hormonal mess inside your body. Really girls, we don't need to add to our current hormonal tsunami! These additives stimulate your body to store more belly fat and encourage cravings.

- **Alcohol.** Drinking alcohol to excess gives only a very temporary illusion of well-being. It will make you fat, make your hot flushes worse, increase the amount you sweat, and increase urinary incontinence. It may lull you to sleep but will disrupt your slumber later. Don't be like the comedienne Henny Youngman, who said: 'When I read about the evils of drinking, I gave up reading.' If you do want a glass of wine, fill the glass with ice cubes to make it last all evening.

- **Caffeine.** Although caffeine may give you that extra boost in the morning, it plays havoc with your body's hormones and how well you sleep at night. Avoid drinking anything that contains caffeine at least eight hours before bedtime because it can take this long for it to clear your system. Many of the symptoms and conditions associated with menopause and post-menopause – hot flushes, difficulty sleeping, vaginal dryness, osteoporosis, lack of absorption of good minerals, lower bone density, slow metabolism and increased risk of heart attacks – are all associated with coffee-drinking. Research conducted by F.E. Norlock and published in the *Journal of the American Medical Women's Association* in 2002 showed that for many who suffer from fibrocystic breasts, giving up coffee will help alleviate breast lumps and pain.

Supplements: what does your body need?

There are so many ongoing debates about whether or not to use vitamin supplements. Medical authorities have vacillated between advising that supplements are a waste of money and even life-threatening to enthusiastically recommending them. After speaking to several health specialists, I have learned that falling oestrogen levels mean that many minerals are not as well absorbed by the body, so some supplements are needed.

The first line of attack for healthy ageing is to get regular exercise and eat a healthy diet of unprocessed foods. Vitamins should never be a substitute for eating well. Taking a high-quality multivitamin every day does not allow you to abstain from eating a healthy diet filled with fresh fruits and vegetables. It should merely supplement what your post-menopausal body cannot get through diet.

Calcium, magnesium and vitamin D

At some point in your life you are going to have to start worrying about your bones. If you haven't put this towards the top of your list, you simply must. Bone loss in the spine begins about two years before you get your last period and continues throughout your life. You can help yourself and fight the laws of nature by exercising regularly and focusing on the strength and resistance exercising discussed in Chapter 3. Nonetheless, ensuring you get enough calcium, magnesium and vitamin D in your daily diet is vital. After menopause, we are less able to absorb these vitamins, so it's a good idea to take a supplement that includes 1200 mg of calcium, 600 mg of magnesium, and 1000 iu (international units) of vitamin D.

CALCIUM

Anyone who studied biology at school knows that calcium is important for strong bones and teeth. What you might not know is that you also require magnesium, vitamin D and zinc to help your body absorb calcium so that it actually stays in your bones.

Good food sources of calcium include soya products, leafy green vegetables, almonds, low-fat or fat-free dairy products (yoghurt, milk, cheese), and tinned salmon or sardines (with oil). Common symptoms of calcium deficiency include nervousness, irritability, insomnia and headaches. Calcium should be taken with meals.

Calcium's many roles

A study done at the National Sleep Foundation concluded that the absence or disturbance of deep or rapid eye movement (REM) sleep is related to calcium deficiency. New research published at the University of Tennessee also found that calcium could be the key nutrient needed to help you lose weight. Columbia University scientists confirm counterintuitive claims that people who are deprived of sleep are more likely to be obese, despite burning calories through tossing and turning. Sleep deprivation reduces levels of leptin, the 'I am full' hormone and raises levels of ghrelin, a hormone that stimulates appetite. Other studies have found that women who increase their daily calcium intake to 1200mg lose weight almost twice as fast as those who do not.

Calcium is important for:

- Building strong and healthy bones and teeth.
- Minimising bone loss and preventing osteoporosis.
- Easing insomnia and aiding muscle relaxation.

- Helping to relieve stress.

- Regulating the heartbeat.

- Supporting the blood-clotting process.

- Encouraging muscle growth and nerve transmission.

- Lowering blood pressure.

- Accelerating metabolism.

MAGNESIUM

Magnesium helps calcium to work better. It is also necessary to:

- Activate the enzymes that metabolise carbohydrates and the amino acids found in protein.

- Regulate body temperature.

- Improve energy levels.

- Lower blood pressure.

- Protect against bone loss.

- Prevent kidney stones.

- Prevent tooth decay (it binds calcium to the enamel).

Natural sources of magnesium include soya beans, halibut, oatmeal, green leafy vegetables, cashews, potatoes and pulses.

VITAMIN D

Vitamin D also helps to make calcium work more efficiently. Historically, nutritionists believed you needed a daily dose of only about 400 iu and that you could get it by being in the sun for 20 minutes a day. In Britain, though, this is virtually impossible, and many of us wear SPF 50 to protect against the sun's harmful (UV) rays. Anyway, it is now believed you need a lot more vitamin D than doctors originally thought. New studies conducted by both the University of California, San Diego, and the Canadian Cancer Society show that boosting the level of vitamin D by as much as five times (1000–2000 iu) could cut the incidence of breast cancer by one-third.

Vitamin D also plays a vital role in:

- Building bone mass.

- Preventing heart disease and many other auto-immune diseases, such as multiple sclerosis, rheumatoid arthritis and diabetes.

- Alleviating high blood pressure and depression.

- Reducing the probability of hip and bone fractures.

- Maintaining muscle strength.

Vitamin D is found naturally in oily fish (salmon, mackerel, tuna, herring and sardines) and eggs.

Other important vitamins and minerals

For optimum health, the body needs a wide range of nutrients, some of them only in trace amounts. The following is a selection of important ones.

VITAMIN E

Vitamin E is a powerful antioxidant that not only helps to turn back the clock, but also prevents some serious degenerative health conditions associated with ageing. It supports healthy skin and protects it from ultraviolet light, protects against bladder cancer, and allows your cells to communicate properly. Recent studies appear to show that vitamin E can also slow down the progression of Alzheimer's disease, but only after it has been diagnosed. As the research is still in its infancy, the vitamin can't yet be definitively recommended for this use.

Vitamin E can be found naturally in nuts (although you would have to eat far too many of them to get the benefit), seeds, olives and their oils, avocados, leafy green vegetables, legumes, blueberries and papaya. The daily recommended amount is 400–800 iu. Vitamin E supplements should not be taken on an empty stomach as they need fats to be absorbed.

B-COMPLEX VITAMINS

B-complex vitamins (which include the whole range of B vitamins) are essential for the health of the nervous system, and can help to prevent anxiety and depression. All are important for energy, good digestion, making and maintaining new cells, and healthy skin, hair and nails.

Vitamin B_{12} maintains healthy nerve cells and makes red blood cells. This vitamin has been receiving a lot of press recently because the results of a seven-year study released by the Karolinska Institute in Sweden showed that high doses of vitamin B_{12} can help to reverse the formation of plaque that cause Alzheimer's disease. Vitamin B_{12} is found in eggs, fish, poultry and other meats. Levels of B_{12} are usually extremely low in older people, so a supplement is needed.

B vitamins are found naturally in wholegrains, animal products, yeast extracts, pulses, nuts, leafy green vegetables and fruit (strawberries, bananas and oranges). A balanced diet, not supplements, is the best way to get vitamin B_{12}.

MEMORY HELPERS

I think it is worth mentioning that there are a few spices that seem to help with memory and tip-of-the-tongue syndrome. Turmeric (an Indian spice) has gained a certain amount of fame in some parts of India where the dementia rates are among the lowest in the world. You can take turmeric either in pill form or in Indian food.

Gingko biloba has become one of the most recommended nutritional supplements in the world. Although it is reputed to improve both concentration and memory, a 2008 study of over 3000 patients (published in the *Journal of the American Medical Association*) found it to be no better than a placebo.

Antioxidant nutrients

Antioxidants are substances that may protect your cells against the effects of free radicals. Free radicals are molecules produced when your body breaks down food, or by environmental exposure to substances such as tobacco smoke, toxic chemicals, excessive sun and radiation. Free radicals can damage cells, and may play a role in heart disease, cancer and other health conditions. They are responsible for many of the degenerative effects of ageing, such as less supple skin and arthritis.

Antioxidants are found in wholegrains and in all the brightly coloured fruits and vegetables. You can find them in the deep red of cherries and tomatoes, the orange of carrots, the yellow of corn, mangoes and saffron; and the blue-purple of blueberries, blackberries and grapes. The most well-known components of food with antioxidant activities are vitamins A, C and E, beta-carotene, the minerals selenium and zinc and, more recently, the compound lycopene, found in tomatoes.

Vitamin C is a powerful antioxidant that encourages healing, builds protection against illness and promotes collagen regeneration (which is why it is sometimes known as the 'anti-wrinkle' vitamin). It also encourages the health of the adrenal glands, which help us to cope with stress.

Nutritious eating for maximum health

The change you make may mean setting more realistic goals, concentrating on eating right and keeping physically active so that you can lead the life you always wanted. If your health or weight interferes with activities you hold dear to you in your everyday life, ultimately you will have to do something about it. Otherwise, you will not be living the life you want to live.

Eating is a major source of pleasure, and we do have to eat to live. Putting the right foods in your mouth will help you transform not only your body, but your mind and spirit. As Hippocrates said, 'Let food be your medicine and medicine your food.'

My top 10 tips

1. Eating well and exercising regularly are the most effective ways to look and feel younger, balance your weight, sleep well, ease menopausal symptoms and experience optimum health on all levels.

2. Cut down on your alcohol intake. Not only is alcohol fattening, but it affects everything from sleep and moods to the intensity of your hot flushes.

3. If you suffer from hot flushes, avoid chocolate, lemon, caffeine, red wine, dried fruit, Cheddar cheese and any foods that contain sodium nitrate (such as processed meats and bacon).

4. Avoid processed foods of any description!

5. Hold the mayo. Always have condiments and dressings on the side. Use dry spices instead of sauces, and stick with mustard, vinegar and dry rubs.

6. Boost your memory through diet – add blueberries, soya, oily fish and flaxseed to your daily menu. Remember when your

mother told you to eat your fish because it was brain food? She wasn't so silly after all. Keep abreast of new studies being released on the memory benefits of vitamins B_{12} and E.

7. If you can't cough, sneeze or laugh without leaking urine, it's best to avoid alcohol, artificial sweeteners, carbonated soft drinks, highly spiced foods and tomatoes. They have all been linked with incontinence in menopause. Remember to do your Kegels (see page 32) any time and anywhere. They will help with incontinence and also keep your vaginal muscles in shape for sex.

8. Up your intake of calcium, magnesium and vitamin D to ease insomnia and other sleep disturbances, while strengthening your bones at the same time. Stay away from alcohol, caffeine and nicotine as they will wake you up in the middle of the night. Avoid chocolate, Coke (Classic and Diet), Pepsi, green tea and hot chocolate as they have surprisingly high amounts of caffeine in them. Eat more foods rich in the amino acid tryptophan (turkey, cheese and milk). The more tryptophan in your brain, the more serotonin too – and serotonin encourages sleep.

9. Keep an accurate food diary. This will help you to monitor two things: the quality of the food you are putting into your body and the amounts of food you are eating. It is easy to forget the late-night snacks of crisps and chocolate. Exactly how many canapés did you have at the last drinks party you went to?

10. Never go on a diet again. Now that you are in the second half of your life, this is a great time to stop thinking about calorie counting and to change the way you think about food. Aim for a healthy, balanced diet with plenty of whole foods. Watch your portion size! Acceptable portion sizes have doubled in the past 20 years. Don't forget your apple cider vinegar. It works at both suppressing appetite and boosting metabolism.

If you are thinking, 'I already know a lot of this stuff', I hope you now understand it better and will apply it to your life in a new way. Doris Lessing said, 'This is what learning is'.

CHAPTER FIVE

Looking your best without plastic surgery

'If you are having plastic surgery out of a fear of ageing, that fear is still going to be seen through your eyes, the windows to your soul.'

Cate Blanchett, actress

D o you remember when you were in your 20s and leaving the house meant running a brush through your hair, making sure that last night's make-up wasn't smeared, throwing on a T-shirt and a pair of jeans, and walking out the door? There was no need to find the magnification mirror to check for new sprouting hairs on your chin; there was no need to see if your grey roots were visible; and there was no need to moisturise your arms and legs so they would look supple and wrinkle-free. Back then, if you remembered to use moisturiser before putting on your make-up, you felt almost virtuous. You really didn't have to think about what clothes you were going to wear because everything looked pretty good.

Now that you are in the second half of your life, looking after yourself can feel like a full-time job. Clothes just don't fit the way they used to, and becoming a magician to hide and disguise your new and growing body parts is an everyday event. The relentless uphill battle with our weight, that begins during the first phase of peri-menopause, as progesterone levels start to fall, will continue for the rest of our lives. Along with the extra kilos, we have wrinkles, grey and thinning hair on the head that coin-cides with unexpected hair growth everywhere else, age spots, a turkey neck, new lines around the eyes and much, much more.

> ❛Wrinkles merely indicate where smiles have been. ❜ *Mark Twain, author*

Of course we all suffer some nostalgia for our youth – the face and bottom we used to have, and the endless energy. But why do some women thrive while others end up depressed and anxious at the prospect of growing old? Some women are annoyed with themselves because they never saw this coming. They view 'the change' as a change of attitude towards them. These women are angry because they don't see themselves as beautiful as they once were. Some women speak of feeling invisible when they walk into a room because they believe they are no longer as desirable. Their value and self-worth is tied up in their youthful looks. They can no longer either consciously or subconsciously trade on their appearance. These same women speak of pharmacology and plastic surgery as their solution to staying young. This is like putting a plaster on a severed artery to stop the bleeding.

The cold reality is that the older we get, the more time it takes to look our best. To the women who are mourning their lost looks I say, 'Stop the self-pity, pay attention, live in the moment and make the necessary changes so you can make the next 40 years the most productive years of your life.'

We can dramatically improve the hand we've been dealt by eating well and exercising regularly. Being fit and healthy is essential to looking and feeling our best. Many women pretend not to care how they look because they have disliked their appearance for so long that they are actually *afraid* to care. If you are one of those women, remember, it is never too late to start making some changes so you can take pride in your appearance.

Be realistic

So what does it mean to stay young? To me it is being fit, staying curious about the world, and being prepared and willing to make the necessary changes to live a life worth living. If staying young to you means having the face of a 35-year-old, you are misguided, will end up disappointed and probably looking ridiculous. We have seen some of the most beautiful women ruin their looks with too much plastic surgery. Remember, even supermodels don't look like super-models in the flesh. In photos they have been airbrushed to death in order to fit the perception of beauty created and perpetuated by the fashion industry. There is an illuminating video entitled *Dove: The Evolution of a Model*. It's worth a look if you think your appearance fails to live up to the high standards set for women today.

I have nothing against plastic surgery, Botox®, fillers and any other facial treatment available to women. If you decide you can afford to and want to have a facelift, eyelid surgery, a neck lift, Botox or collagen injections, autologous fat implants, Hylaform®, Restylane® or any of the other injectable treat-ments, then do it. But take care. You need to find a great, board-certified cosmetic surgeon who believes that less is more and has ideally been recommended by a friend who had a good result. There is nothing that will age a woman more than a plastic surgeon with a heavy hand.

If you are not happy with how your face looks, but don't want injectables or to go under the knife, there are other procedures to try, such as chemical peels, radio frequency and laser skin-resurfacing treatments. You could even opt for having eyelash or hair extensions. These beauty enhancers may be just what you need to give your appearance the added lift you have been looking for.

Varicose veins or spider veins qualify as a bona fide health concern. For spider veins, a simple laser procedure or salt injec-tions performed in a doctor's surgery will give you your desired result. If you have varicose veins, they will simply get worse without treatment, and pose a serious health issue, so go to a doctor and get them seen to.

True beauty comes from within

I am, however, concerned when this obsession with changing our appearance gets in the way of deeper self-respect and the belief that there are truly wonderful and inspiring years left to live. How many times have you heard, 'How can others love you if you don't love yourself'? It's often repeated because it is true. Turning ourselves into superficial cosmetic wrecks prevents us from believing in and loving ourselves. To be beautiful, we need to stay mentally and physically active to ensure that we have the *joie de vivre* needed to rediscover and empower the best in ourselves. Being unable to walk without pain, or face each day without the energy needed to continue living life how we want to, is a lot scarier than a few wrinkles and age spots.

Cosmetic surgery has given women the superficial chance for 50 to be the new 35. What is worrying is watching women and the media obsessing with how to repair the surface. We know too many women who make increasing numbers of subtle changes to their appearance – the more they try to fix it, the worse it becomes. It is an accident waiting to happen – where beauty collides with creepy in the overwhelming pursuit of good looks.

Developing an obsession with superficial beauty can stand in the way of self-awareness and even self-liking. It goes without saying that we would rather not wrinkle, but this doesn't even compare on the Richter scale to living a life in pain because we didn't work on taking care of what matters beneath our skin.

When you can readily list all of the things that you dislike about your body and face, you are probably feeling unattractive and dissatisfied with other parts of your life. Will Botox and other beauty potions make you look in the mirror and feel beautiful again? Are you the fairest of them all? Nothing bores a man faster than a woman obsessed by her ageing appearance. When the late-night conversation comes back to 'Do I look old?' or 'Do I look as old as her?' or 'Do I look fat?' your partner, if he loves you, will begin to worry *for* you. If your relationship is already on shaky ground, I am afraid all the injections and surgery available to you will not be enough to make you feel beautiful again or put you back on to terra firma.

We all know true beauty comes from within: our personality, our intellect, our creativity, our nurturing spirit, our directness, our ability to take on new challenges, and our unique energy.

Beauty from the inside out

There are plenty of ways to look your best and have skin that radiates good health and happiness. Women who like themselves and feel comfortable in their own skin are the ones who captivate the entire room. A confident woman – a woman who is interested in the world around her, has purpose and passion, makes others feel comfortable, smiles and laughs easily – is the one that both men and women would categorise as beautiful.

Yes, of course your metabolism is slowing down, you can't read a newspaper without reading glasses, you probably get up at least once in the night to use the toilet, and you are noticing a lot more wrinkles around your eyes, forehead and mouth. It is probably your ageing skin that is bothering you the most at this point. You will need to learn to take care of your skin and accept the inevitable changes that occur with age.

Making peace with yourself

The key to being at peace with your appearance is to look your best by making the most of what you have. Regular exercise and eating well will help you to feel beautiful inside and out. The magic will come from the change in you. This doesn't mean cosmetic surgery to change your appearance, but celebrating your best features and using some tried-and-tested tricks to improve the ones with which you are not quite so happy with.

Must-haves

The following items are essential for the post-menopausal woman. They will help to make you look your best every day, and you will wonder how you ever survived without them.

Power pants

As far as I'm concerned, power pants are the number one fashion 'must-haves' for the second half of your life. If you don't know what they are, Google 'slimming shapewear' now, and you'll see the wide variety of options available to transform your figure. Power pants reconfigure any flab and smooth you into a sleeker, slimmer shape. They can instantly make you look 4kg thinner, and give you added confidence to wear the figure-hugging dress that has been hanging in your closet for the past five years.

Shapewear comes in all shapes and sizes. As well as the traditional stomach, thigh and hip shapewear, there is now a 'cami' that slims your midriff, waistline and tummy, and even a whole dress that sucks you in from shoulders to mid-thigh. Once you own one of these seemingly magical garments, you won't be able to live without it. Whatever you choose, well-fitting underwear is important, as you'll not only feel more comfortable, but you'll make the most of the shape you have. It's worth noting that peri-menopausal women are prone to yeast infections, so cotton is a good choice, although it is not the sexiest.

Wearing a good bra

It is important to have a bra that is comfortable and fits well. Several studies have concluded that at least 70 per cent of women wear the wrong-sized bra, which can cause not only back and posture problems, but also damage the fragile ligaments of the breast. It's hard to believe that when bras were first developed in the 1920s, they were designed simply to provide support for a woman's breasts in order to prevent sagging and backache. Today bras play a variety of roles, and you can choose your bra according to what you want it to do. Some women want to look bustier, while others want to minimise their size. The most important thing is to choose a bra that gives your breasts the shape and appearance you want, and then to make sure it is the right size. Most good lingerie shops and department stores have professional bra-fitters, who will take a series of measurements to ensure that you are wearing the correct cup and band size.

It's worth noting that some brands fit differently to others, so try on lots to find the one that feels comfortable, looks great and fits perfectly. A perfect fit is achieved when the centre of the bra, between your breasts, sits firmly on your chest, the cups hold your breasts without any overspill or ruching of the fabric, and the band is comfortable on the loosest setting.

Tweezers

Let's face it, tweezing is not simply necessary to ensure that your eyebrows are well shaped and tidy. You also need them to deal with the *other* hair sprouting on your chin, cheeks, moustache and neck. Unwanted facial hair is caused by the decrease in oestrogen. During and after menopause, facial hair becomes more masculine and is known as 'terminal' hair, which is longer, coarser and darker.

If you are tempted to save time and shave off this new hair growth, don't. Designer stubble is not a good look at any age. Laser, threading and electrolysis can take care of the problem in the short term, but these treatments are expensive. Waxing is another option, and while it can be effective in the short term, it requires regular treatments to keep hair growth at bay. Whatever method you choose, it's worth investing in a good set of tweezers to remove any stray hairs that appear. Look for professional-quality, 100 per cent stainless-steel tweezers, which are longer lasting and will not rust when cleaned. The most popular are those with a slanted tip because they give more precision and can be used for most tweezing needs.

Magnification mirror

Alongside your trusty tweezers, you'll do well to invest in a good magnification mirror. Mirrors come in magnifications of 1, 3, 5, 7 and 10, which is effectively the number of times your image is magnified. Make sure you have some natural daylight to give you a proper view of your problem hairs. Magnification mirrors let you isolate even the finest hair for precise, easy tweezing.

Facial hair bleach

Although I am a big fan of waxing above my lip and threading my eyebrow hairs, I don't seem to have enough time to go to a salon or spa to get it done as often as I need to. In between professional treatments I rely on facial hair bleach to make sure my moustache does not look like I have just escaped from the circus. There are lots of brands available at the chemist. Waxing strips are also available for emergency clean-ups.

Hair colour

Anyone who tells you that you look better and younger being grey or 'salt-and-pepper' is not a friend you can trust when it comes to beauty. If you are lucky enough to go white, it can be beautiful and elegant. But as far as I'm concerned, you should not even think about letting yourself go grey until you are at least 75! Grey hair ages you overnight, no matter how youthful your skin and body look.

If you are simply touching up your roots between salon visits, buy a product that is for roots only. Leave it on for a good 20 minutes, even if it says 10! If you are colouring your whole head, leave the product on for an additional five or 10 minutes. Grey hair is usually very colour-resistant and stubborn. If you do colour your hair at home, it's worth paying a visit to a good colourist every few months for some highlights as your hair can end up looking flat, dull and lifeless without the occasional lift. A little expert guidance from professionals, who are used to matching colour to skin tone, can be invaluable.

Choose a colour carefully. If you are brunette, for example, and don't want to look like Morticia from the Addams Family, select a colour that is at least a shade or two lighter than your natural colour. As your skin ages, it becomes paler or more sallow, so lighter shades can look better. The opposite is true for blondes. Ultra-blonde hair is very ageing after 50. Go for warmer shades that approach *café au lait*. Even Madonna recently went for a caramel hue. If that seems too conservative, add a few ultra-blonde highlights – but just a few!

Hair mascara

This is an easy way to hide grey roots that appear between colouring sessions. It is applied like mascara to grey roots and will give you an extra week or so before you'll have to colour again. There are also hair crayons that can blend re-growth or grey along your hairline, but I would recommend the mascara.

Shampoo and conditioner

Lower levels of oestrogen cause the hair on your head to thin dramatically during and after menopause. Hair tends to be dryer, thinner and more brittle than it was before 'the change'.

It is essential that you purchase a good shampoo and the best-quality conditioner you can afford so that you can make the most of the hair you have left. Using a moisturising treatment every one or two weeks will also make a huge difference to how young your hair looks and feels. If you are sleeping alone, drenching your hair in olive oil and wrapping it in plastic apparently does wonders to restore lost lustre. If your hair loss is particularly bad, there are treatments available that should be discussed with your doctor.

Essential blow-dry tools

A hair-dryer, four round hairbrushes, hair serum and hairspray – yes, you need all of them! I enjoy washing my hair and I've now mastered a few tricks that make it look like I've been to the salon for a wash and blow-dry. After I wash and condition my hair, I put a little hair serum through the ends to make my hair silky and soft.

Blow-drying is an art form unto itself. I have found the only way to make hair look like it has been professionally dried is to use three or four round brushes, all curling my hair at once while I am blow-drying. Find the brush size that works for your hair length and buy four of them. They will lift your hair and give it the shape and bounce you want – all in a fraction of the time it takes to blow-dry your hair using one brush.

Hairspray will help to keep your hair from losing its lift just as you arrive wherever you need to be.

A great haircut

As we age, the hair on our scalp thins and it seems to move to our chin! We must make the most out of the hair we have left. To encourage hair regrowth, make sure you are eating enough omega-3 fatty acids by including salmon, sardines, herring or mackerel in your diet two or three times a week, and add two tablespoons of ground flaxseed to your cereal or salad.

Finding a great stylist who can cut and blow-dry your hair in a way that makes you feel and look wonderful is like finding a plumber who will come out and fix your washing machine on a Sunday. They become important people in your life. If you are not happy with your hair, ask a friend whose hair always looks good to recommend her stylist. Having a great haircut and blow-dry will definitely improve the way you look, no matter how you may be feeling.

Good-quality skincare products

With the reduction of oestrogen in the body, collagen and elastin are reduced and the skin becomes thinner, dryer and less supple. Skin needs special attention to ensure that lost water is replaced through moisturiser, and it needs to be kept clean to ensure that the products you use work effectively. Remember to cleanse, tone and moisturise (in that order) every morning and night before bedtime, and support this regime by eating a healthy diet that contains the nutrients important for skin health (vitamins A, D, C and E in particular), and getting plenty of exercise to help your circulation and encourage healthier-looking skin.

Did your mother use Pond's cold cream to cleanse her face? After experimenting with dozens of brands, I have come to the conclusion that Pond's is the best, least expensive and most effective way to cleanse my face. However, when it comes to moisturisers and eye creams, it's worth experimenting a little. Not only will you need to find the ones that work best for your individual skin, but you will need to spend as much as you can afford to get something that is truly effective. Make sure your daily moisturiser contains sunscreen (look for an SPF factor of at least 15) to protect your skin from the ageing effects of the sun. In fact, do yourself a favour and stay out of the sun, getting vitamin D from your food and a vitamin supplement instead.

Make-up 101

Cosmetic companies employ make-up artists to show you how to use their products and to help you realise what best enhances your features so that ultimately you will buy their products. The artists know what they are doing, and you get to sample their products properly before deciding if they are worth buying. You should definitely take advantage of this fun and free service – though describing it as 'free' is definitely questionable. As you transform from the girl next door into a catwalk model in about 20 minutes, the 'free' make-up lesson could end up with you buying the products that have been used, which could cost you hundreds of pounds.

Tinted moisturiser and foundation

Good-quality products will make your skin look fresh and glowing. In the second half of life, the skin is more susceptible to thread veins and uneven pigmentation. For the most natural coverage, choose a tinted moisturiser, which not only plumps up your skin and protects it from the sun (they usually contain SPF coverage), but gives you a natural glow. Make sure you ask the make-up artists to try a few different products and colours before you decide to make your purchase. When I look exhausted and need an extra boost, I use both a tinted moisturiser and then a foundation on top. Dust a neutral mineral face powder over your moisturiser or foundation to avoid that horrible shiny, glow-in-the-dark look. Remember, though, by far the best way to get a youthful glow is to exercise or, better still, have sex before going out for the evening.

Electric toothbrush

Looking after your teeth and gums becomes increasingly important as the years pass. Not only are you more susceptible to osteoporosis due to your changing hormones, but you are also more susceptible to tooth decay and swollen and bleeding gums.

Teeth can become overcrowded as the shape and size of your jaw change. If you don't own an electric toothbrush, you should go out and buy one because it will stimulate your gums and help to address the areas where plaque and bacteria tend to build up. Don't forget to floss too – twice a day if you can – to encourage good oral health. The best floss is made from Gore-Tex, which glides easily between the teeth. Don't forget to tell your dentist exactly where you are in your menopausal journey. He or she may be able to tell you a lot about your bones by looking at your teeth.

Whitening toothpaste

Tea, coffee and just about everything you eat can stain your teeth as you get older, largely due to thinning and more porous enamel. Whitening toothpastes can remove unsightly stains, and also make your teeth look years younger. There are many brands available, including some for sensitive teeth, and others that help to remineralise the tooth enamel. If you can afford it, get your teeth whitened professionally. Otherwise, a more affordable solution is tooth-whitening strips and kits that you can buy at the supermarket or your local chemist. Feeling happy about how your teeth look will give you the confidence to smile. People look at your face and sense your state of mind long before they are checking out anything else about you.

Nail varnish

I don't know why, but women seem to be genetically pro-grammed to have their nails painted beautiful reds, pinks and purples. It makes us feel complete to look down and see our nails perfectly shaped and polished.

Post-menopausal women tend to suffer from dry and brittle nails, so it is a good idea to give them one week a month without polish so they can 'breathe'. Rub oil and lotion into them, avoid harsh chemicals and don't overuse polish or hardeners.

Did you know?

The natural colour and state of your nails could be a sign of possible health problems.

- Dark nails signal a B_{12} deficiency.
- Pale or white nails could be a sign of anaemia or problems with the kidneys/liver.
- Red nails could be a sign of heart disease.
- Pink and white nails point to kidney disease.
- Grey nail-beds are symptomatic of conditions such as arthritis, glaucoma, cardio diseases and excessive malnutrition.
- Yellow nail-beds suggest possible liver disorders, diabetes, lymphatic diseases or chronic bronchitis.

Footcare products

A pumice stone, nail clippers and a foot file are essential to keep your feet and toes looking their best. During the peri- and post-menopausal years, the skin on the palms of the hands and soles of the feet becomes thicker. This can cause painful cracking and splitting, so you'll need to pay particular attention to these areas. To remove dead and thick skin or calluses from your feet, use a pumice stone or skin file every time you take a shower or a bath. Make your own exfoliating, sea-salt scrub by mixing any coarse salt or brown sugar with olive oil to create a paste. Rub it on your feet, rinse and then use the pumice stone or foot file, repeating if necessary to get a good, smooth finish. After your final rinse, apply a foot cream to moisturise. Not only will your feet be more comfortable, but they'll look great too.

Body moisturiser

During and after menopause, the skin on your body is affected every bit as much as your face, and you'll experience pigmentation issues, dryness, sagging and wrinkles where you least expect them. Take time to treat your body with a good moisturiser, paying particular attention to your arms and legs, especially in summer, when a product containing sunscreen should be used. To keep your skin supple and silky, use baby oil in the bath. It doesn't cost a fortune and you can pour in as much as you want and make it feel like a guilty pleasure. There are various inexpensive moisturisers available for your body, from E45 to petroleum jelly, which is particularly effective on your feet. Moisturising is absolutely essential for any post-menopausal woman.

Perfume

Wearing perfume is a bit like wearing make-up. It gives us a boost because we like the way we smell when we wear it. Find a scent that you like and stick with it so that it becomes something like a 'signature' scent. It should be an extension of who you are, and should ignite that sixth sense in your husband or partner. The scent will remind him that it is you he wants to be with.

Reading glasses

Mid-life, at around 45 years of age, is the time when your eyes start changing. The lenses begin hardening, leading to the need for reading glasses. Hormonal fluctuations can also cause problems with eyesight. The problem with reading glasses is that you can never find a pair when you need them. If you are anything like me, you'll end up buying at least a dozen pairs and leaving one in every room of your home, not to mention two in the car to read the A to Z. If money is tight, you can purchase inexpensive glasses from a pharmacy. Take along a book and experiment with the different strengths to see which makes reading easiest for you. Alternatively, you can visit an optometrist, who will give you prescription reading glasses that will be made and fitted just for you. In this case, one really good pair can be firmly attached on a chain around your neck.

Sunglasses

Besides doing what they were invented to do – reduce glare and protect the eyes from harmful UV rays – sunglasses can cover up the fact that you haven't slept well or you are having a bad day. What's more, if you suffer from dry, itchy eyes during your menopausal years, you can wear sunglasses to protect them from the wind. Headaches and migraines caused by bright lights are also common during 'the change', and sunglasses can help prevent these too. Aim to get the pair that fits the size of your face, looks great and gives you a bit of glamour. Designer sunglasses have become something of a fashion must-have, but for women over 50, they are simply a must. When your eyes are puffy and the skin around them is creased from sleeping, no one will ever guess if you disguise them with a good pair of sunglasses. Polarised are best.

Handbags

For women, purchasing a new handbag is mood-altering. It doesn't matter how many kilos we may be over our ideal weight, a brand new handbag makes us forget those extra kilos. A handbag ranks as one of the ultimate fashion accessories. You can transform any daytime outfit just by changing your handbag to a glamorous evening clutch. A beautiful handbag is an *objet d'art* – in fact, Lulu Guinness's handbags are part of a permanent collection at London's Victoria & Albert Museum. Need I say more? What about buying shoes to match?

Black is not just for mourning

The colour black is one of the greatest gifts to women over the age of 50. It's a slimming colour and masks a multitude of sins. What's more, there is a certain dignity and elegance that black proffers. I think there are a few black items that every woman needs:

- **Opaque black tights.** I love these, and my teenage girls live in them! Not only will they help to make your legs look longer and thinner, but they'll hide any flaws, lumps and bumps as well. Go for something with a denier of at least 40, so there is no sign of skin showing through. You can purchase tights containing Lycra and aloe, and even tights that claim to alleviate cellulite. Wear them with **black leather boots** – either ankle- or knee-high – with a little heel. They will definitely help to make your legs look longer and thinner.

- **A little black dress (LBD)** is a must for every wardrobe. You need to start collecting LBDs just as you would wonderful shells on the beach. They should be as simple as possible, making it easy to dress them up or down with the proper accessories. If you have fantastic legs, your dress should really come down to just above the kneecaps. Watch heads turn as you walk into the room.

- **Black pencil skirts and straight-leg black trousers and jeans.** Wearing black on the biggest part of your body will create the illusion that you are slimmer than you actually are. Avoid wearing busy patterns on the bottom half of your body.

- **Black or dark navy fitted blazer** that falls to the hip. This looks great over a white, tailored, button-down shirt. Remember, you don't have to button your jacket, so make sure it fits you across the shoulders. Better to buy it one size smaller if necessary, as it will look great but just doesn't button.

- **Black workout clothes.** Putting on flattering workout clothes will help you to get yourself to the gym, park or yoga studio. As a general rule, black on black is the most flattering.

- **Black swimsuit.** For most women over the age of 50, buying a swimsuit is about as much fun as sticking needles in their eyes. The first rule is Lycra and the second rule is a one-piece. A good one-piece, solid black bathing suit should hold everything in, make you look thinner and cover the most difficult part of a post-menopausal figure – your midsection or tummy.

Bicycle

Yes, you read that right! If it's good enough for the prime minister and the Mayor of London, it is definitely good enough for you. In fact, it is the coolest accessory for anyone who is trying to get fit and keep green. Make sure you get a detachable basket for all your shopping, and a helmet too. Cycling is terrific aerobic exercise. You will burn fat, tone your muscles and speed up your metabolism. What could possibly be better than that?

My top 10 tips

1. Buy clothes that fit properly and that will instantly make you look thinner. Wearing clothes that are too tight so you can tell your friends you can squeeze into a size 12 will make you look bigger than you are, and emphasise your lumps and bumps. On the other hand, wearing baggy clothes will make you look heavier than you are, and if you think for a second you are fooling anyone about what is beneath that outfit, you are sadly mistaken.

2. If you are thick around the middle but have thin legs, wear a hip-length flowing top or tunic. Team it with a black skirt that comes to just above the knee, black opaque tights and black boots to emphasise those great legs and cleverly hide your expanding waistline.

3. If you are less than 5 feet 6 inches tall, wear a small, preferably chunky, heel as it is easier to walk in them and there is less risk of falling over. Platform shoes or boots with heels give you additional height, plus the appearance of being thinner. Dark-coloured shoes balance whatever is going on above the knee.

4. If you have toned arms, wear sleeveless dresses or shirts. If you are lucky enough to have a small waist, wear a belt to highlight it.

5. If you have a beautiful long neck, wear a necklace that shows it off. Virtually every high-street retailer sells costume jewellery, and you don't need to be a high earner to afford it. It will dress your neck and keep people looking at you above the waist.

6. If you have nice breasts and an unfreckled smooth chest (no sun damage), wear clothing with a slightly lower neckline, but be careful about showing too much cleavage. It can be ageing.

7. Accessorise, accessorise and then accessorise some more. Accessories can make or break a look. You can take the dress you wore to work and morph it into the most wonderful evening outfit by changing your jewellery and attaching a feathered clip or silk flower to your hair. Find accessories to create an identity that belongs only to you. Old clothes can become instantly fashionable again by teaming them with a vintage brooch, a chunky necklace or a pair of chandelier earrings.

8. Summer love should not be with the sun. Use a sunscreen with a high protection factor to protect against ultraviolet rays, and tell your daughters to start using it now too. Sun damage makes anyone look 5–10 years older.

9. If you smoke, give it up. Smoking ages the skin even faster than the sun because nicotine stops the blood flow to the capillaries. The increased health risks are not worth it.

10. As a friend of mine says, 'Clothes look best on a well-toned body.' Make sure you exercise almost every day of the week and eat a nutritious diet. Start today and become stronger, more energetic and happier. There is no magic potion or pill except exercise and eating well to make you feel beautiful inside and out.

The style you choose is an expression of who you are and a reflection of how you feel about yourself. Style is not about how much money you have or buying designer clothes, but believing that if you buy a dress from a charity shop or a flea market it can be as chic and beautiful as anything that will give your wallet a battering. Style is something unique to *you*.

How we look and dress tells the outside world how we view life: are we optimistic and full of hope or filled with despair? I know there will be days when you think, 'Who is this woman in the mirror staring back at me?' If you are over 50 and haven't figured out how to make the most of what you have and how to hide what needs hiding, you'd better have the body of Jerry Hall or the wit of Ruby Wax. Otherwise, review these top tips and figure out how to look your best.

Getting older really can mean getting better. Once you have solved the problem of how to dress to emphasise your positives, remember to take that power of positive thinking and internalise it too. This will help you build your new equilibrium for a productive, happy and creative second half of your life.

CHAPTER SIX

Your changing brain
A different kind of passion

'Our deepest fear is not that we are inadequate. Our deepest fear is that we are powerful beyond measure. It is our light, not our darkness, that frightens us most. We ask ourselves, "Who am I to be brilliant, gorgeous, talented and famous?" Actually, who are you not to be?'

Nelson Mandela

If you thought of yourself as a well-balanced, reasonably measured and optimistic person, the years of peri-menopause may well have given you reason to pause. The uncertainty of how your brain was going to react to any given situation was the start of your transformation. Although you did not feel as if you were moving forward, these changes laid the foundation for your brain to transform into this last phase of development, when you have the renewed desire, energy and focus to be the person you always wanted to be.

You might believe that this transformation goes hand-in-hand with the changes happening in your own life, such as children growing up or leaving home. However, do not under-estimate how your changing hormones levels are affecting you. Oestrogen is a key element in brain function, and a part of its signalling system. In fact, studies have shown that oestrogen and progesterone are not just sex hormones that influence ovulation and reproduction; these hormones also affect a large number of cognitive functions.

The mind controls a complete spectrum of emotions, as well as our imagination and desires. During the years leading up to and after menopause, our brain is asking us to rediscover the best in ourselves. The voice of 'How can I find more meaning in my life?' becomes the voice that leads you to rediscovering your passions – and rediscovering the best in yourself.

According to Dr Louann Brizendine, author of *The Female Brain*, there is another hormone responsible for this change – oxytocin – the connecting and tending hormone. 'The brain's circuits don't change all that much in the mature female brain, but the high test fuel – oestrogen – that ignited them and pumped up the neurochemicals and oxytocin in the past has eased off.' This biological truth is a powerful stimulus for the road ahead and the road back to yourself. 'One of the great mysteries to women at this age and to the men around them is how these changes affect their thoughts, feelings and the functioning of their brains'.

Do you have less fear about trying to achieve some of the goals you are setting for yourself? Could this second wind, sometimes referred to as 'post-menopausal zest', give you the desire and courage to explore and reach your true potential?

Redefining passion

Your changing hormones will be the catalyst to cultivate dormant passions and embrace life with a renewed vigour. This is your time to use your emotional, physical, mental and sometimes spiritual energy to find the essence of what you truly enjoy. This is what passion is. Passion is the energy that supports us to engage in and focus on the thing we do for ourselves to make us feel fulfilled.

All one has to do is look around and see how women are transforming themselves by making passion a bigger part of their everyday lives. They are setting up farmers' markets in their towns and villages; starting book clubs and theatre clubs; learning new languages; joining their local choir; going back to college to train as teachers, lawyers, writers, psychotherapists, architects, doctors; setting up businesses on the web; learning to play the piano; and enrolling in life-drawing and design classes. Women are rediscovering their passions with a vision of what they think their tomorrow can be – and adding their determination and drive to make *their* lives better.

I have spoken with so many women who are beginning again. They are rediscovering old passions or finding new ones, and re-engaging with themselves and their community in a new way. The voices of fear, failure and self-doubt that have held them back from living the life they want have become quieter. Shakespeare said, 'Doubt is a thief that often makes us fear to tread where we may have won.' Post-menopausal women are hitting their stride and tasting success.

So how can you set about your own journey to find or rediscover your passions? There are a few key questions you need to be able to answer:

- What brings a smile to your face? What excites you? Maybe it's some part of your job or a hobby you loved in the past but just haven't had enough time to pursue?

- Do you have a secret dream? To ride your bicycle across France? To learn how to cook Japanese food? To sing in a choir? To learn how to play tennis or golf? To learn another language? To read all the classics?

- What are you good at? Are you a good connector of people? Is organising a pleasure rather than a chore? Do you enjoy teaching others?

- Do you now have enough time to pursue your passion(s)? Can you make the time?

- Are you willing to take the small steps to pursue what could bring you enormous pleasure in the second half of your adult life? Is the fear of failure holding you back from making this commitment to yourself that will transform your life?

You only have to pause and think how fast the last 30 years have flown by to realise that the next three decades will pass in the blink of an eye. By making passion part of your daily life, your brain and thought patterns will start to grow again, along with your curiosity and interests. Life will once again seem like a big adventure.

Find the person you left behind

By the time your child embarks on his or her first school trip, you will know that change is just around the corner and your dependant 10-year-old is only a few years away from discovering their own independent life. They are just beginning to use their 'wings' to fly out of the warm nest that was their entire world. Short hops away from the nest become longer flights. Don't think for a moment that your children will always want to be with you and need you. They won't, and if you aren't prepared for this fact, it will hit you like a ton of bricks. If you gave up certain hobbies or sublimated other interests for the good of the family, now is your time to start again and find the person you left behind.

Before you start to make a list of all the things you would like to do to fill your life with passion, begin by visualising what will make you want to *anticipate* the next 30 or 40 years.

Proper preparation and a first-rate attitude are needed so that you don't wake up one morning and realise you have an empty house and no interests or passions. You need to start thinking and planning when your *kids* start to think for themselves. It is important to your development and theirs.

Don't expect to instantly leap into a new way of life. Old habits are hard to shake, and you will undoubtedly experience an awkward stage of transition between the carer you were and the new vibrant woman you are on the verge of becoming. It takes courage to re-engage and start again where you left off. Fear can be the greatest obstacle in moving forward and making the most of your abilities, and as we hit 50, and even 70 or 80, new fears rear their ugly heads.

We fear how we will age, we fear feeling useless, we fear the possibility of death, either our own or of those close to us, we fear being alone and acting and sounding old. We know what old sounds like. I used to be afraid to ask my mother how she was feeling because 20 minutes later I was still getting a blow-by-blow description of every ache and pain in every muscle and joint in her body. Add to this a pessimism about the future, then your spirit, personality, curiosity and outlook on life can become tainted and your world small.

Taking care of your mind by reigniting passion will give you more energy and desire to enjoy your post-menopausal life. Our state of mind directly affects how we feel about ourselves, the way our body looks and behaves. When we are feeling depressed or stressed, our body responds in kind and we become more susceptible to bugs and illnesses – anything to slow down, stay in bed and get some tea, love and sympathy. When we are feeling on top of the world, the last thing we want to do is find ourselves ill in bed, and the odds are heavily in our favour that we won't be. *Mens sana in corpore sano* – a sound mind in a sound body.

The vicious cycle of stress

Stress negatively affects the way we think and view the world, and how our brain functions. How you decide to tackle and manage it will definitely have an effect on the outcome of your menopausal journey and the rest of your life.

Here is how the vicious hormonal cycle of stress and irritability plays itself out. Our adrenal glands produce cortisol.

Cortisol is the stress hormone. When cortisol is high, it blocks oestrogen from reaching our cells. When less oestrogen reaches the cells, our serotonin levels fall. Serotonin is a hormone that acts as a neurotransmitter, transmitting messages to our nerve cells. Changes in the level of serotonin in the brain can affect our moods, causing anxiety, depression, panic, insomnia, headaches, migraines and a reduced interest in sex. In a nutshell, low serotonin makes us irritable, short-tempered and depressed.

When serotonin drops, another hormone and neurotransmitter is released in the brain: norepinephrine. This is responsible for giving us a pounding heart and more hot flushes, and it wakens us in the middle of the night with the fear that we are having a heart attack. All of this makes life more stressful. So guess what happens next? Our cortisol levels get higher, blocking oestrogen from our core cells, which subsequently encourages serotonin levels to fall further. It's worth noting that caffeine, alcohol, cigarettes, sugar and exposure to artificial light on a television or computer screen can also negatively affect your body's serotonin levels.

With so many stress triggers, we can't be certain if we are clinically depressed or simply experiencing yet another symptom of 'the change'. We don't consider ourselves to be happy; we find little pleasure in life. We may also drink more alcohol, become anxious and tired a lot of the time. And this vicious cycle keeps on spinning. The irony is that although we may feel alone, there is a huge crowd of women experiencing exactly the same thing.

Is there a way to naturally increase our levels of serotonin? Yes. Exercise daily, eat properly, use your brain and rediscover your gifts, share those gifts with friends, family and your community, and remember to have fun.

The power of yes

When you have a passion, you know why you are here on earth. Cultivating a passion is an expression of who we are and what we care about. You must try to push aside your doubts and fear of failure that prevent you from saying yes to exploring what-ever nourishes your mind, body and spirit. Take some risks and the rewards will be huge.

By pursuing your passions you will be giving yourself the chance for greater happiness. Like ageing, happiness is not a matter of luck. Is the glass half-empty or half-full? My mother-in-law lived and breathed the half-full attitude her whole life, and happiness and health followed her everywhere. The choice is yours.

Remember to say the word 'yes'. If someone asks you to organise a charity sale, say yes. If someone asks you to join a book group, say yes. You may find yourself transformed from just saying yes to doing the organising and the asking. You must make the leap from saying no to yes because your mental state will change every time you give a positive answer. Say yes to socialising. Say yes to employment. Say yes to new opportunities.

Use it or lose it

Keeping your mind active by cultivating passions is directly correlated with a longer lifespan and the regeneration of brain cells. Dr Marion Diamond, a neuroscientist at the University of California at Berkeley, and author of more than 100 research articles and books confirms, 'New nerve growth in the brain can be created even in people as old as 90, simply by introducing new challenges in the environment. Our challenge is to learn ways to keep the brain functioning at an optimum level for a lifetime.' She goes on to say that we need to 'change our negative attitudes toward ageing for ourselves and for others'. Use it or lose it!

THE SECOND HALF OF YOUR LIFE

Dr Lawrence C. Katz is co-author of *Keep Your Brain Alive*. He says, 'The mental decline most people experience is not due to the steady death of nerve cells. Rather, it is the atrophy of connections between nerve cells in the brain.' He believes that routine behaviours, many of which are almost subconscious and require little brain power, contribute to such atrophy. He has developed a system that he calls 'neurobics' – exercises to stimulate the brain – which is based on two principles: experiencing the unexpected and enlisting the aid of all our senses during the course of the day. Even something as simple as sitting on a park bench, looking around you and then, without looking again, writing a list of everything you just saw can keep the mind alive.

Key lifestyle changes to keep your brain energised

1. Eat more fibre and less sugar.
2. Grease the cogs of your own wheels by eating more omega-3 oils (see page 112 for sources).
3. Colour your world by putting on your plate bright orange, purple and red fruits and vegetables.
4. Mind your ABCs, but especially your Bs – i.e. B-complex vitamins, and in particular B_{12}.
5. Get enough sleep.
6. Stay connected to family and friends.
7. Use it or lose it.
8. Relax and give yourself time to unwind.
9. Watch your weight.
10. Eat lean, clean and green.

Are you listening?

Being able to listen and respond to the questions your post-menopausal mind is asking you will help to propel this change in you. Who am I? What do I need? What is my body asking me to do? What is my brain asking me to do? Do I have interests that will help me feel fulfilled?

We must pay more attention to the things we love and make sure they bring meaning to our lives. You may now have the time to explore a new passion – the love of your grandchildren. Every person I know who has grandchildren says the same thing: 'Grandchildren are the best! There is nothing better in the world.' How wonderful to spend time with these little people you love completely, yet have the pleasure of returning them to their parents at the end of a visit. You can read to them, introduce them to the joy of words, bake cakes, grow vegetables and make each time special. It is a pure, uncomplicated and enriching love. This love is a passion.

Another important part of this rediscovery is learning to be content spending time alone. Solo time is a reality of getting older, so you need to make it something you enjoy. Learning to get in touch with the silence within yourself while you live with your children, husband or partner will help you to value the time you spend alone. If you are not comfortable with your own company, you are going to spend a lot of time wanting and hoping to be somewhere else.

There is a fine balance between being content doing solo pursuits and actively engaging in your life outside the home. For many women, the need to reconnect with old friends and make new friends through common interests becomes a life force. When you meet other people who share your passion, meaningful and deep friendships will follow. Worlds expand and life becomes more interesting.

Be social and put yourself in situations where you can make new connections. Make socialising like a second job, and one you excel at. Besides creating new connections, meaning and friendships in the second half of your life, research has shown that rediscovering your passions will help to protect the brain from dementia and slow its progression.

You know what makes us old? Idleness, overeating, sitting in front of a television for days on end, a lack of curiosity and being alone. Women like to connect – we were designed to connect. We physically *need* other people around us to share experiences and just *talk*. So push yourself to get out there and be with people.

Men vs. women: Mars vs. Venus

Incredible as it may seem, there is a biochemical reason why women want to talk and connect. When women talk to each other, the 'cuddling' hormone, oxytocin, is released in the brain. Oxytocin blocks stress hormones, so we actually feel better. Interestingly, although oxytocin is released in both men and women when we talk, it actually blocks testosterone in men. In other words, it makes them feel less manly, less sexual and even moody. The good news is that as men grow older, they care less about the things affected by testosterone and we become much more alike.

Throughout history, women have endured persecution and even death because the greatest male philosophers, religious leaders and thinkers of the day had no understanding of what made women act and think the way they did. We know men and women think differently. Some of the differences are related to the way we were raised and the roles and tasks our parents asked us to do as children. Other differences are the product of hundreds of thousands of years of genetic and evolutionary behaviour and, ultimately, because hormones determine how we think.

According to scientists, it is our hormones that support not only lactation but our bonding and nurturing behaviour. According to Deborah Blum, author of *Sex on the Brain*, this is the reason why 'boys get intense about Lego and girls do not'. If men had oestrogen instead of testosterone, they would not be from Mars, and we would all be living on Venus together. We can't ignore the fact that men and women are created differently and therefore think differently. What is intriguing is how men have successfully controlled and dictated how women should think and behave for thousands of years.

The rise of the Tupperware culture

It was only 60 years ago that Western women believed their lives should be defined by the roles of wife and mother. In fact, at the turn of the last century, US President Grover Cleveland proclaimed, 'Sensible and responsible women do not want to vote. The relative positions to be assumed by man and woman in the working out of our civilisation were assigned long ago by a higher intelligence than ours.'

Society offered women only two choices: housewife and mother (happiness) or career and spinsterhood (tragedy). The media was very effective in convincing women that the path to fulfilment was to renounce their own goals and dreams, and to dedicate themselves to a life of narrow domesticity. What every woman thought she wanted – and believed she needed – was a husband with a good job, at least two healthy children, a lovely home in the suburbs with a driveway, a dishwasher and a shiny new washing machine.

This, of course, led to the belief that you could consume your way to happiness, with Valium ('mother's little helper') and the Tupperware party. Tupperware became a phenomenon because it was one of the few acceptable and available outlets for our mothers and grandmothers to connect with other women, earn a little money, and be an entrepreneur within the confines of preserving the myth that homemaking was everything.

The most brilliant and beautiful young women of the 1950s went to university as a means of securing a husband, not to prepare themselves for a career. Women in that era knew it was not smart to appear too intelligent. It would scare away the boys. No man wanted to share his life with a woman who would threaten him in any way.

The goal of university was to graduate with a solitaire diamond on your left ring finger, have invitations printed, and choose a beautiful white wedding gown.

The history of female inferiority

Almost 100 years earlier, in 1859, Charles Darwin published his groundbreaking theory of evolution in his book *On the Origin of Species*. His model of evolution put women where they had been for thousands of years – below men in the pecking order, and distinctly inferior. According to Darwin, men needed logic and reason to survive, and women – well, they simply needed a womb and breasts to have and care for children. Darwin believed that a woman's worth was in her reproductive organs. Leading scientists, philosophers and evolutionists supported his theory by comparing human brain size to argue that women were simply less intelligent than men. If it was smaller, they believed, it had to be inferior.

When it comes to the size of a man's penis, we know smaller does not mean inferior. But the prevailing wisdom of the day suggested that women's smaller, (the Victorians called it 'the missing 5 ounces of the female brain'), less-evolved brains were not equipped to think logically or garner knowledge, and that our smaller bodies were not capable of physical exercise. With little or no physical exertion – and few mental challenges – the average Victorian woman had no interest in anything, including sex. As Hera Cook observes in her book *The Long Sexual Revolution*, a frigid and repressed woman was considered the 'perfect ideal wife' for a Victorian man. Although scientists believed that women were controlled by their reproductive organs, the female body was little more than a pair of ovaries and a receptacle for semen.

Freud never understood women

Next on the scene was the psychotherapist Sigmund Freud, whose brilliant theories about the subconscious mind kept women from fulfilling their potential for two generations. He disguised his lack of understanding of the female brain with terms such as 'penis envy' and 'super-ego'. This prevented women from seizing new opportunities in the post-Victorian era. The uncritical acceptance of Freud's doctrines in both America and Europe made it virtually impossible for women to question this new psychology. Any expression of self-fulfilment was viewed as penis envy. How could women question the unconscious mind and the psychology of truth and think they could possibly come out on top? Freud reigned supreme.

Freud's premise was quite simple: get rid of your suppressed envy and a neurotic desire to be equal and you can find sexual fulfilment by affirming your natural inferiority. Women should be ruled by men, and the limitless subservience of women was taken for granted by Freud. He was the new spiritual leader and his words were the new gospel. Although he was zealous in his views about women, he admitted that 'the great question that has never been answered ... despite my 30 years of research into the feminine soul ... what does a woman want?'

Back to domesticity

By the mid-1940s, educated and accomplished women began publishing books of their own that had a tremendous effect on the lives and minds of female society. When *The Psychology of Women* by Helene Deutsch was published in 1944, it was considered the most comprehensive analysis of women's development at that time. Deutsch reconfirmed and fully endorsed Freud's doctrines: any expression of self-fulfilment could be equated with penis envy. Sexual pleasure could be achieved only when a woman renounced all goals of her own.

Femininity equalled passivity and dependence; masculinity equalled activity.

Three years later, in 1947, the overnight bestseller *The Modern Woman: The Lost Sex,* by psychoanalyst Marynia Farnham and sociologist Ferdinand Lundberg called for widespread psychoanalysis, education and government subsidies to restore women to their traditional domestic roles. It pushed for women to believe they needed to be completely dedicated to their children and husband to have an identity in society, thereby negating the progress women had made during the war years by working outside the home and fostering a sense of worth apart from the family. Filled with pages of psychoanalytic theory, it simply reiterated what women had been told for hundreds of years – they should return home and do what they were created to do: make babies.

It was only in the mid-1950s that scientists began to consider that a woman's brain could be linked to her menstrual cycle, and thus the radical concept of pre-menstrual syndrome (PMS) was introduced to the scientific community.

This concept didn't reach centre-stage until the 1970s. British physician Katharina Dalton wrote a bestselling book called *Once a Month*, in which she cited lovely, nice wives becoming surly and obnoxious once a month. She campaigned for PMS awareness, suggesting that fluctuating hormones caused personality transformation. This far-reaching idea – that changes in women's hormone levels were linked to how we behave and view the world during certain days of the month – started to change the way women thought about themselves and the way men thought about women. It was the beginning of real change and understanding for both sexes.

Could history repeat itself?

When America sneezes, the rest of the world catches a cold. This is usually said in terms of the United States' leadership in finance, fashion, technology, the stock market and higher thought. The rise of Sarah Palin, the Tea Party she hosts and the doctrines she and her followers espouse – anti-choice, abstention as a form of birth control (we saw how well it worked with her own daughter, Bristol), anti-masturbation (who could be against this?), and their questionable stance on equal pay for equal work – must give women around the world cause for concern. Could what Palin refers to as 'conservative feminism' spread to the rest of the world? Do the American women who support her believe that she is a hockey mom and devoted wife who just happens to be the leading Republican nominee for the office of President of the United States? Who is fooling whom?

Firing up your brain cells

The second half of your life is about choice and change. If, as you grow older, you want to stay acting and feeling young, you will need to choose to continue improving your mind by staying interested, engaged, committed, connected and active. Just as you need to exercise your body, you will need to train your brain to stop atrophy setting in. To achieve this, Dr Lawrence Katz recommends engaging our senses and 'stimulating ourselves mentally'. A mentally stimulating life has a positive effect on all aspects of our cognitive function and memory, and reduces the chances of suffering from Alzheimer's or dementia. Even simple things, like doing the daily crossword puzzle or practising your mental arithmetic by not using a calculator, can help. Think about what you would like to learn about and put yourself in a place where you can do just that.

Matching brain span to lifespan

How can we match 'brain span' to lifespan so that we do not just live for a long time, but live fully? According to co-founder and chief scientific officer of Posit Science, Dr Michael Merzenich, 'Recent studies have shown that the brain retains its natural plasticity throughout life. Engaging neuroplasticity in adulthood requires intensive, repetitive brain exercise. It's probably not surprising to you that brain exercises can help keep the brain fit: "use it or lose it" has inspired many people to do crossword puzzles and other activities to stay sharp.'

Learning to perform new and challenging activities can engage the brain's natural plasticity to make positive changes. Merzenich believes there is limited value in working at a game or exercise that you can perform without paying close attention. It is important always to strive to take it up a notch to a higher and more demanding level, where you re-engage the brain's learning machinery.

It's on the tip of my tongue

As we get older, many of us suffer from memory lapses or poor memory recall. These are the 'senior moments' that haunt all of us. It is scary. When we can't remember the names of people we worked with 10 years ago, the name of the restaurant where we ate only a month ago, the name of a play we saw last week, or why we went to the supermarket, we fear the worst. The good news is that this is not dementia or Alzheimer's. Those diseases really have more to do with having trouble remembering *how* to get to the local supermarket, the names of your close friends and feelings of disorientation.

Many of us believe our brains are not functioning well during the years of peri-menopause. Hormones, and the havoc they wreak on our sleep, definitely play a leading role. If our brains are microprocessors, many of us feel the need for an upgrade, a faster chip. By challenging ourselves to use our brains more, we can help to stem the tide of the 'tip of the tongue' syndrome. Play little memory games with yourself. Go to the supermarket without a shopping list and see how many items you remember to bring home. You will be surprised how good your memory is when it needs to be; if not, you will see how many items you bring back that you already have in your refrigerator. Eat foods rich in omega-3 oils to help keep the brain working the way it should. Research has shown that exercise and a good diet play huge roles in how the brain works and retains information later in life.

As we get older, there can be a temptation to isolate ourselves and narrow our lives, which not only encourages the type of atrophy that Katz describes, but also leads to loneliness, inertia and a lack of opportunities to connect and create the passions we need to make our lives meaningful. When you are on your own, keep up with what is happening in the world. Read a newspaper every day. Stay current. If you don't already have an email or Facebook account, ask your children or grandchildren to show you how to set one up. It is a great way to communicate with them and reconnect with old friends. Buy a Kindle or an iPad and read the books you have always wanted to read in digital form. When you have reignited the passions that have always been important to you, you will keep yourself open to discovering new ones.

Embracing an attitude of growing through lifelong learning means not only keeping your mind active, but creating opportunities to meet new people who share similar interests with you. You might create a new career opportunity. You might even make a new connection with someone who becomes a wonderful friend, companion or life partner. Here are just a few ideas to keep your brain firing on all cylinders:

- Learn how to play a musical instrument, or improve your ability to play something you learned as a child.

- Learn how to play bridge, chess or backgammon. If you don't have anyone to keep you company, you can play these games on a computer.

- Go back to school to learn about something you always wanted to know more about or to help start the career you always dreamed of having.

- Start a new hobby: crafts, painting, biking, photography, rambling or bird-watching.

- Join a current events club – or an investment group, where you can use your spare pennies to play the stock market.

- Put your maths O level to good use, and take control of your finances. Work out the best place to save or invest your money, and how to make your earnings or pension go further.

- Learn a foreign language, and then travel to that country with a friend or your partner.

- Join a theatre, cinema or arts club. If there isn't one locally, start one!

- Play tennis for your local club or join a tennis group at your level of play.

- Stay informed about the world – read magazines and newspapers. Challenge yourself by reading magazines or books you wouldn't normally read – something outside the realms of what is familiar to you: science, car mechanics, art history.

- Write an article for your local newspaper about something that inspires you – or write a letter to the editor.

- Join a book group. Indulging yourself in books and reading will keep your mind stimulated while creating new social connections.

- Read about a wide range of subjects. Your local library is a good place to start.

- Learn how to use an iPod and download podcasts to listen to new music and books.

- Take a computer class, and if you don't own a computer, make it first on your list of must-have purchases. Use email and Facebook to communicate with your children, grandchildren, school and university friends. It is the connections you create and re-create that will keep you happy and stimulated.

- Plan a holiday to a place you have never been before, and learn all about its history prior to going. If you don't have someone to go with, book with a university or museum travel group.

- Take cooking classes, read recipe books and try out new dishes on friends and family.

- Take up a new exercise or join your local team so you can play competitive sports.

- Master your daily newspaper's sudoku or crossword puzzle.

By cultivating at least one passion, and hopefully more than one, you will be providing yourself with the opportunity to keep learning, stay curious and become involved. Most of the activities that create new connections, meaning and friendships in this part of our life cost very little money, but bring a wealth of benefits. Resuscitating old passions and cultivating new ones create a back-drop to help you to continue to thrive for the rest of your life.

My top 10 tips

This is my prescription for health and happiness. Stick it on your refrigerator and live by it.

1. Continue to dream up new projects and adventures. Adrian Zecha (born 1933), founder of the Aman chain of resorts, says he stays young by keeping his dreams vivid, his passions strong, his mind and body active and his purpose great. He says, 'I will become old when my dreams become smaller than my memories.'

2. Plan ahead. Have activities to which you look forward.

3. There is no need ever to retire. Just continue to reinvent yourself. Slowing down doesn't mean giving up – ever.

4. Read more and expand your interests. Have an opinion. A unique outlook shared makes everyone think more. The more you know, the more interesting you are to yourself and others.

5. Give people in your life more than they expect and do it happily. Look for the best in people.

6. Spend some time with people you love every day, but also spend some time alone. Try to avoid too much introspection – it usually leads to depression.

7. Do something that connects you with your body for at least 30 minutes every day. (See Chapter 3, if you are in doubt!)

8. By cultivating and having passion and interest in your life, you will have a more positive outlook and attitude about life and the people you come in contact with. Light attracts light. Smile when you pick up the phone. The person who has called you will hear the smile in your voice.

9. Cultivate your passions in order to create new meaning and connections in your life. Pain is mysterious. The best way to fight pain is to stay busy with the things that give meaning to you. Make an effort to meet new people by actively engaging in the things you enjoy doing. It will expose you to people, and possibly new friends, you would not have met otherwise.

10. Remember the power of positive thinking. You *can* do anything you want to do.

The secret of growing old *well* and ensuring the best years are still to come is to keep improving your mind by staying interested, engaged and actively committed to what matters to you. Now is the time to make sense of the years you have already lived and make some small changes to give your life passion, purpose and meaning.

CHAPTER SEVEN

Finding purpose
The gift of rediscovery

'Service is the rent we pay to be living. It is the very purpose of life and not something you do in your spare time.'

Marian Wright Edelman, president and founder of the Children's Defense Fund

If somebody told me when I was 35 that I was going to live to be 96 years old, I might have said, 'That's nice. I hope I will still be able to walk and talk at the same time.'

I never thought of ageing as the beginning of another adventure, a chance to continue to grow and deepen, rather than remain stagnant. The gift of menopause and the years after are not just about being alive, but seeing and engaging with the world in a new way. This is a time when a woman can give birth to herself.

Passion is about you and the things you do for yourself. Purpose is completely different. Purpose gives passion an anchor. Purpose is an expression of who you are, your core values and what is important to you. It is about making a difference and living a life of meaning. Helping others: family, friends and your community. Purpose is about using your special talent, gift or ability in a way that will benefit others. Purpose defines *why* we are on this planet.

Of course, what give us purpose may change at different points in our life. For the first half of our adult life a career or taking care of our family may fulfil our sense of purpose, but when the children grow up and leave home, we may feel we have lost it. We may also get purpose from the work we do and the goals we have set for ourselves. Sometimes it is the process of getting there that gives us purpose, and once we have achieved our goals, we may begin to struggle to find the sense of fulfilment we once had.

Of course, purpose for each of us will be different. It could mean service to our community, supporting worthy causes we care passionately about, helping out with grandchildren, reconnecting with nature, helping people we meet, or simply being the best we can be. Purpose comes by connecting to the greater good and expanding our circle of caring. It is listening to our calling and what we are here on earth to do.

Now, in the second half of life, our brain is asking us to reconnect with the world in new ways. After a few years of feeling as if we are living in darkness it really is, 'Nice house, lights are on and welcome home!' This discovery gives each of us another chance to find the best in ourselves and to feel more purposeful than we have at any time before. Living with purpose will become the biggest driving force in our life.

The great equaliser

There are defining moments for everyone. For me, one was when I first became a mother and I had overwhelming feelings of admiration and respect as I watched other mothers calmly deal with crying, screaming and unruly children as if they were Mary Poppins. Their race, religion or educational background didn't matter. I wanted to learn from them. Motherhood was a first great equaliser.

How we choose to grow old is the next and final big equaliser. We are all in the same boat again: coping with aged parents who need to be looked after, missing the children who no longer live with us, struggling with unwelcome health issues, learning to cope with fluctuating hormones and other issues of ageing, being married to or living with the same person for a long time – or divorced from ones who didn't value us, or whom we stopped loving.

Our new, deep feelings of admiration and respect are directed to the women who are using the second half of their life to become the people they always thought they would or could be. Our new role models are the women who want to be recognised for *how* they live and the things they *do*, not the number of years they have lived. Having a purpose greater than yourself will give you a renewed sense of well-being. This will make one of the biggest differences between healthy and unhealthy ageing.

You can finally put to good use the trait that has annoyed your husband and friends all these years – your single-mindedness. Use your stubbornness to formulate and stick with a plan to create a life worth living. If you haven't been a particularly single-minded person, become stubborn. Stay connected to friends, family and your community so that when you aren't feeling on top of the world, you have a sense that you matter.

Find the real you

Having a purpose greater than yourself will give you a renewed sense of self-esteem. By ensuring through regular exercise that you have the strength to greet each day with the vitality you need to make your life worth living, you will give yourself the chance to stay connected to the world of which you want to be a part. If you can't walk unaided, or every step you take causes pain, you won't be able to confront each day with the energy needed to make the second half of your life meaningful. This could be the difference between waiting to live and waiting to die.

Human beings were not created to live alone – we used to live in packs, hunt in packs and sleep in packs. Solitary confinement, exile and enforced isolation have been the most severe of punishments through the ages. Isolation can cause mysterious diseases to appear and make worse any pain you experience. In fact, isolation and feeling separated from your family and community are among the main causes of premature ageing.

Everyone's goals will be different, but anchoring them with a cause you care about will give you both a sense of satisfaction and purpose. Caring for the people you love, helping the greater good, stimulating your brain by continuing to learn and offering your time and expertise to help others in any way you can will help you rediscover the best parts of yourself. This is your time to make what you care about most a much bigger part of your life.

> ❝Life begets life. Energy creates energy. It is by spending oneself that one becomes rich.❞
>
> *Sarah Bernhardt, French actress*

Giving back

The reasons why people choose to volunteer are as varied as the opportunities that exist. Some people volunteer because they believe it is their duty to give back: they can make a difference, give others less fortunate a chance, and initiate change by believing passionately in the cause. Some volunteer because a friend is involved, and some decide that giving time and a talent can be more valuable to an organisation than just giving money. Volunteering is the first step in your search for purpose.

The quickest and easiest way to begin learning about the size and scope of the various charities that exist and what they do is to start with the 'Do-it' website (www.do-it.org.uk). At any one time, 'Do-it' has over 1 million volunteer opportunities. It also has one of the easiest websites to navigate and offers the most comprehensive answers to any question you might have about volunteering.

Another excellent resource is 'Volunteering England' (www.

volunteering.org.uk), a countrywide network of volunteer centres dedicated to finding opportunities in your local area. The Charity Commission also has a helpful website (www.charity-commission. gov.uk). Every registered charity must be listed with this organisation.

Once you have a clearer idea of what is out there, ask yourself the following questions:

- How much time do you realistically have to give in a week or a month?

- What skills do you have to offer?

- What do you want from your volunteering experience?

- What sector of the volunteer world do you care about most? Do you care most about sports and underprivileged children? Sustainability in Africa? Aids? A local museum or theatre? Mentoring children? Breast cancer? Osteoporosis?

- Would a large or small organisation suit your personality and skill sets?

Once you have decided you want to volunteer, spend some time giving this process further thought. Do you have an interest about which you feel passionately? If the answer is 'yes', you will need a plan. If the answer is 'no', you will need to start formulating a strategy. Visit a few organisations, ask questions and meet with other volunteers. If they offer training or orientation sessions, use this opportunity to assess where you might fit in. Organisations have needs, and even if you are giving your time for free, their needs must be fulfilled.

Ultimately, volunteering gives you an opportunity to get involved and engaged, meet other people with similar interests, and help others. It will give your life new meaning.

'Meaning' is one of those overused terms. For many, it has to do with the inner and spiritual self. However, 'meaning' can also be outward – learning, developing and applying knowledge to the world around you. It involves looking, learning and finally attaching and taking ownership of something more important than yourself. It gives value to your life.

The magic of giving

Women who give their time to a cause they care about believe this is the best investment they have ever made. One woman told me, 'Whatever I gave in terms of my time, expertise or introductions came back to me in different ways at least by double or triple. Giving my time to charity transformed my life.' This is part of the magic of giving. It is one of the best ways to create community, meet new people and make new friends and acquaintances of all ages and backgrounds who share your sense of purpose. It keeps building on itself. You are needed. You are appreciated. You are connected. You know where you belong. Giving your time to help others in any way you can will inspire you and those around you.

Many post-menopausal women I interviewed found themselves in a whole new stage of creativity and productivity through discovering purpose. When I started volunteering at the Donmar Warehouse theatre, it brought me closer to my childhood dream of being an actress and working in the theatre. My time there opened up other opportunities in the theatre world. I started working with the Mousetrap Theatre Project, a wonderful charity that gives less-privileged children the opportunity to see the best theatre in London. Combining passion with purpose can transform the life you live. Another woman said giving her time to charity was 'a gift to her soul'. Supporting an organisation you believe in, will provide you with a purpose which creates a framework to help you flourish.

Can money buy you happiness? Apparently the answer is 'yes', as long as you spend the money on someone else. According to new research, giving other people as little as £5 can lead to increased well-being for the giver.

Creating and seizing opportunities

In his life changing book *The Seven Habits of Highly Effective People*, Stephen Covey says that part of being proactive is to envision what you want and how to get it. He writes, 'Being proactive means being responsible for our own lives; taking responsibility for our own lives; taking initiative; acting instead of being acted upon. Proactivity empowers us to create circumstances.'

Psychotherapist and author Susie Orbach warns: 'You may need to try a few things before your interests begin to deepen. Having a purpose requires discipline to sustain those difficulties and not give up.'

Some of the angst that plagued you in the first half of your life will take a back seat. You like who you are. You worry less about how people view you. Researchers from Stony Brook University in New York found, after interviewing 340,000 American men and women between the ages of 18 and 85, worry tends to tail off when we hit 50.

The great philosopher Ralph Waldo Emerson once wrote, 'All life is an experiment. The more experiments you make the better.' So keep trying and putting yourself out there. You will eventually find what works for you. If you haven't been able to find "the" something that inspires you yet, keep trying new things, and for now, put the end result towards the back of your mind.

In the beginning, it doesn't matter *what* you do. By offering your time and lending a hand in any way you can, you will not only start enriching your life through helping others, but when you begin to become involved it has a curious multiplying effect on your life. By actively supporting the causes you care about, you are combining passion with purpose and creating life opportunities for yourself.

If you are naturally shy, remember the *yes* word. Say *yes* to everything. As you rediscover a purpose in your life, you put yourself in a position to share it with people who enjoy doing the same things that you do. A common connection creates a natural bond. It becomes easier to relax and open yourself up when you share a mutual purpose. Together we have a lot of living to do.

Say 'yes' even if you are skeptical. Don't think the opportunity isn't big or important enough, or that it won't lead to anything. Don't worry about the fact that your abilities may not be fully challenged. Take what is on offer and make it yours. As you rediscover your purpose and make that purpose a part of your life, it will become as big or important as you want it to be. This part of your life is about you and what you make of it.

Can we have it all?

Our definition of 'having it all' has definitely changed over the years. When we were in our 30s we thought having it all meant a great job, a nice husband and a couple of kids. In our 40s we figured out that we did not need to prove – to ourselves, our mothers, our husbands or our friends – that we could be the world's greatest juggler. If we were lucky, we started to lay the foundations for the rest of our lives. A friend told me, 'I knew this time of my life was coming, and I knew that if I didn't make some dramatic changes in my 40s, the rest of my life would be spent wishing I had. That is my advice to other women: start planning in your early 40s for the rest of your life.'

A place in the world is not something we *find,* but a life we *create.* We will achieve our rightful place when we live a life filled with purpose; when we commit ourselves to something larger than ourselves. When we were younger, we spent our days juggling our busy and demanding lives. Now is our time to live a life building purpose and cultivating passions.

Having purpose takes a determination and energy to nurture a life dream along with managing the realities of everyday life. Of course, as the children grow up and leave home, it becomes easier to be clearer about what is important to *you* and to make these things a priority. You finally have the time to immerse yourself in all the interests that you once had but were too busy to do anything about.

Everything in this book is about fixing the parts of your life that aren't working so you can stay focused on what you can control – the parts that will change how you grow old, feel about yourself and see the world. Unearthing your dreams and capabilities, redefining your deepest hopes and desires, and identifying your needs will make this stage the greatest learning and discovery period of your life. As feminist and writer Betty Friedan once said, 'Ageing is not lost youth but a new "stage" of opportunity and strength.' Start learning your lines because you finally have the script to make the second half of life your best half.

My top 10 tips

1.   Think about what interests you. Take those interests and make them important to you. It will be inspiring and enriching to you and those around you.

2.   Remember, you are a repository of wisdom. Continue to speak to the next generation about what defines a meaningful life because your experiences are not only meaningful to you but to others.

3.   Learn new skills. Education and mental stimulation correlate to a longer lifespan and reduce the risk of Alzheimer's and dementia.

4. Mental activity will do the same for your brain as physical activity does for your body. Stay curious and open minded.

5. You are never too old to try something new, and you are never too old to let your dreams become a reality. Do not resist change. Continue to create opportunities for your future.

6. Put someone else's needs first. It will go a long way to making others happy, and ultimately create a happy and fulfilling life for you. As Mark Twain said, 'Whoever is happy will make others happy too.'

7. A hobby can turn into a life's purpose and give deep meaning to your life. When you live a life filled with passion, you create the life you choose to live.

8. Be courageous and say 'yes' to giving your time to help others. The rewards of taking this risk could be potentially huge changing not just your life, but the lives of those around you.

9. Invest the time to discover your life's purpose. It will give you a reason for getting out of bed each morning.

10. Focus on the areas of life that are important to you, and you will find that great things happen to you because of you.

By rediscovering purpose in your life, your mind will start to grow again, along with your passion and vitality. As we know, one of the biggest obstacles to living life to the fullest is our attitude. By volunteering and giving back, you create a wonderful basis on which to thrive through all your post-menopausal years. When you find a purpose greater than yourself, you put yourself in the best place to rediscover the best in you.

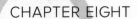

CHAPTER EIGHT

Sex

The naked truth

'Women might be able to fake orgasms. But men can fake whole relationships.'

Sharon Stone, actress

When a man thinks about sexual gratification, he is biologically programmed to get his penis inside a woman and ejaculate. According to science, the grand plan is called the 'continuation of the species'. This involves making the minimum investment for the maximum return to ensure the survival of one's genes. Somewhere along the line, men got to have their cake and eat it too.

It was only 60 years ago that women believed they were abnormal, frigid and somehow derelict in their duties as a good wife if they did not reinforce the androcentric model of sex: foreplay (getting a man ready for sex), penetration and male orgasm.

Can you imagine the frustration our mothers, grandmothers and previous generations of women endured as they were made to think they were failures and sexually hung up because they could not have an orgasm from penetrative sex?

Speaking of sex

It's not as easy as you might think to get women to talk about their sex lives. I believe there is a dichotomy between what women believe they should say and what really happens in a long and well-established marriage or relationship. I sent out 300 separate email surveys to women over the age of 50, asking them to elaborate on their sex lives: the number of times a month they had sex; if sex had changed while going through the peri-menopause; what changes they experienced, e.g. intensity of orgasm or pain during intercourse; and what, if any, treatments they were on – HRT, localised oestrogen treatment (Premarin cream, Estring or Vagifem) or other lubrication to help with vaginal dryness. Only seven replied – and only one responded with direct answers to my questions. The other six were a variation on, 'I will get back to you' or 'Would you like to have a cup of tea and chat about it?'

I think that both peri- and post-menopausal women don't like to talk about their sex lives because they feel anxious about the subject and worry that they are the only ones experiencing any problems. Are we covering up for ourselves or the men in our lives? You might remember that the word 'menopause' comes from the Greek *mens*, meaning 'monthly' and *pausis*, meaning 'cessation'. Many women seem to believe that it can be more literally translated, reflecting their views of sex during this period of their lives: give 'men a pause'.

Sex, lies and menopause

When I went to gather more information about sex and the older woman from a respected gynaecologist she started by saying, 'I suppose you will be writing about how women rediscover their sexuality after menopause.' When I expressed my surprise, as this view was so different from what I was hearing from ordinary women, she then asked, 'Oh, so you are going to write the truth?'

Encouraging women to open up was more than interesting – it was fascinating. Most married post-menopausal women who had been married for over 15 years would begin the interview by saying that they had sex maybe once or twice a week. I would then ask if they had noticed any change since going through the menopause. Did they initiate sex or was it their partner? Interestingly, the number of times they had sexual intercourse went from once or twice a week to once every couple of weeks. Occasionally, the answer was once or twice a year. More than one woman said she loved her husband, but sex was just not what they did any more; she had not had sex for at least two years. Another woman asked, 'Does anybody have sex with their husband after menopause?'

One married woman, who had not had her period for just over three years, responded candidly, 'The only part of my body that is getting thinner is the lining of my vagina! My urge to have sex has evaporated into thin air. No matter how much I love my husband – and I do – if it hurts, I am not exactly fantasising about my next sexual encounter.'

Another interviewee said, 'Sure I have sex with my husband, but it is something I feel I have to do. I have sex because he wants to, or I am trying to convince him to take me somewhere special. It's a trade-off – a blow-job for a holiday in Majorca. I am very happy to do this to keep my marriage stable. I definitely don't have a sex drive any more.'

A fantastically beautiful and intelligent 52-year-old woman disclosed that her husband had told her that her vagina would close up if she didn't have regular sex – the use it or lose it philosophy. There is definitely some truth to this, but she was having lubrication issues. She asked if he said this because they were not having enough sex.

I had heard somewhere that women actually develop a stronger sex drive and start to enjoy sex more than ever after they go through menopause. Christiane Northrup even wrote a whole book called *The Secret Pleasures of Menopause*. The thinking is that there is a lot less to worry about in the second half of life – no need for contraception, no kids around, fewer financial pressures and lower inhibitions – thus allowing couples to embark on a sexual renaissance. This wasn't exactly what I discovered from my research. What I unearthed is that most newly divorced or single women still hoping to find Mr Right find the same desire and sexual intensity that they did in their youths with a new partner, but peri- and post-menopausal women who were in long-term relationships did not experience the 'pleasures beyond their wildest dreams scenario' when it came to sex.

One newly single woman in her late 50s, who recently left her husband for a much younger man said, 'I thought I was all dried up because I didn't have sex for well over eight years with my husband. But now I am having sex regularly and enjoying it more than ever.' Another new divorcee said she could finally shake her strict Catholic upbringing and view sex as a bit of fun without looking for commitment.

I found a lot of single women in their 50s and 60s making this kind of comment. What I couldn't find was anyone who had been married for a long time to support the 'secret pleasures of sex after menopause' theory. It was like searching for the Holy Grail!

I could find plenty of very happy, long-married couples who lived and travelled together and had a great time. Yes, many had sex regularly, but nobody was talking about sex getting better. So you can imagine my excitement when I went to a lunch and sat next to a woman who told me that after she went through menopause, a sexual desire unlike anything she had ever experienced was awakened. When she was not teaching her midday cooking classes at home, she would call her husband to come home and have sex. She said that all she could think about was sex. Nobody else had said anything like this, so a few weeks later I phoned her to double-check a few facts. I started by asking her when she had stopped getting her periods.

She said, 'No, I still get my periods. I am as regular as clock-work. Why? Does something happen to your sex drive after they stop?'

Who needs an unreliable friend?

Maybe you are one of the lucky ones and your sex drive is as strong as ever. For most women, though, hormones work against them. As the hormones that historically defined our sexuality start to disappear, sex – which we could always depend to keep us connected – became an unreliable and untrustwor-thy friend. Whereas in the past it had 'greased the wheels', reconnected you to your partner and made you both happy, it suddenly became confusing. You woke up one morning and didn't like your husband's smell or the way he kissed. You stopped wanting to be intimate. You found it more difficult to have an orgasm. What turned you on before did not have the same desired result.

There is no question that the physical effects of menopause and lower hormone levels can take their toll on your sex life, even if you previously always enjoyed it and were the one initi-ating it. This is because the vagina becomes physically smaller due to a lack of oestrogen and your sex drive decreases due to a drop in testosterone.

To have to withstand a pain similar to losing your virginity every night is not something anyone wants to sign up for. And if sex has been painful for a while, you and your partner will both have an emotional and mental block about lovemaking, regardless of how much you love each other and want to make love.

The urge to have sex was always bubbling just under the surface in our younger years and worked perfectly during the years we wanted to become pregnant. As one peri-menopausal woman said quite openly, 'Women want sex all the time when they want to make babies. We all know a woman's libido is at its absolute strongest when she wants to get pregnant. We think about sex morning, noon and night.' Getting home from work early and doing nothing but spending the whole night in bed making love is the making of a perfect evening. Well, sort of. At the age of 35, I remember being told that if I wanted to get pregnant, I had to keep my legs in the air for 20 minutes after having sex. I'm sure this particular routine was not exactly a turn-on for my husband but he definitely wasn't complaining.

In the heat of a woman's biological need to make babies, your husband may be thinking, 'Not tonight, dear!' If we are being completely honest, after the man you have chosen has successfully impregnated you with his seed and you have all the children you want, the urge to have sex with him isn't quite the same.

Mix in the precipitous drop in hormones that occurs during the years leading up to menopause and it is perfectly natural for women to go off the idea of sex. Hormones, or lack of them, are the real culprit here. Dwindling supplies of oestrogen, progesterone and testosterone will definitely play havoc with your sex drive and the way you enjoy sex. Many very real and unpleasant physical changes also take place, which can lead to:

- Loss of elasticity and thinning of the vaginal tissue.

- Reduction in the blood supply to the vagina, which can make it too dry for comfortable sex.

- Decrease in the amount of natural lubrication.

- Decrease in the size of the clitoral, vulval and labial tissues.

- Smaller cervix, uterus and ovaries.

- Lower libido/sex drive: orgasms become less intense and the anticipation before an orgasm decreases.

- Increased vaginal itching and irritation.

- Higher risk of bladder infections after sex.

If anyone tells you that any of the symptoms described above are in your head and unrelated to menopause and decreasing hormones, you must realise that they don't know what they are talking about. If someone has the nerve to suggest that you need to see a psychiatrist or sex therapist, or insinuates that your marriage is in trouble because you are either not interested in sex or have pain during intercourse, know that what you are experiencing is completely normal and the medical profession actually has a cure for it.

More bells and whistles

Although sexual problems are difficult to talk about it can be extremely beneficial and important to discuss them, as you could actually pick up an idea or two to help you sort out whatever you and your partner may be struggling with. Virtually all of the women I interviewed agreed that there was a definite need for a few more bells and whistles to help make sex more pleasurable. Run, don't walk, to your local pharmacy and purchase an over-the-counter, water-based lubricant, such as KY jelly, Sylk or Astroglide. If sex has been painful for a while, buy Replens MD, which lasts up to three days. Actually, buy both – they could solve your problem in 10 seconds. If you are allergic to glycerine, there are non-glycerine products available, such as Aqualube and Hydrasmooth. Another possible solution for treating dryness and pain during intercourse is to insert a vitamin E capsule into your vagina. There is no need to break open the capsule; the pH of your body will do the job.

You might feel a bit awkward at first about using these products but, believe me, your partner will be thrilled. It will quickly become a part of your foreplay routine. Do not use Vaseline, as it provides a wonderful home for bacterial growth. Also, if you are still menstruating, obviously you can still get pregnant (duh!) and Vaseline can weaken the latex used in condoms. Stick with a water-based lubricant.

Do your best not to imagine the worst when your doctor tries unsuccessfully to put a speculum inside you and tells you that your vagina has atrophied. It might conjure up images of a weakened, shrivelled vagina that is withering away, but help is at hand. While lubricants and gels are great for lubrication, vaginal atrophy may require something more. Your doctor may prescribe a vaginal oestrogen cream, which can reverse thinning and encourage the health of your vaginal tissues. You may also be offered an oestrogen ring, which is inserted into your vagina and slowly releases oestrogen in the area that needs it most. Rings will continue to work for about three months, but release a low dosage of oestrogen, thus having little impact on hot flushes or other symptoms of menopause. An oestrogen pessary can also be used. This is effectively a capsule or gel-like tablet that is placed in your vagina to release oestrogen to the affected area.

Some doctors will automatically recommend systemic HRT because they view it as an all-in-one solution to menopausal problems. It can help to ease painful intercourse and reduce other menopausal symptoms, such as osteoporosis, heart disease, hot flushes and night sweats, but you will need to weigh up the risks and benefits of HRT before embarking upon this type of treatment. See page 42 for further information.

Good vibrations

For thousands of years, women were expected to reach orgasm through coitus and were discouraged from masturbating on the grounds that it would impair their health.

The vaginal orgasm was promoted by Sigmund Freud, the father of psychoanalysis. He laid the groundwork for the next two generations of women to abandon the clitoris's sexual primacy to the vagina's. According to Freud, mature women had vaginal orgasms, while clitoral orgasms were experienced by psychosexually immature women. This gave men licence to be selfish and left a majority of women sexually frustrated and wondering what was wrong with them.

Given this historical backdrop, the invention of the best sex toy for women, the electro-mechanical vibrator, is worth exploring. The electric vibrator, invented in 1883 by a British physician, Dr Joseph Mortimer Granville, solved a problem that plagued the medical profession from the time of Hippocrates until the 1920s: namely, how to effectively and efficiently treat the most commonly diagnosed ailment in women – hysteria. According to Rachel Maines, author of *The Technology of Orgasm*, massaging female patients to orgasm was the only known cure for treating this 'disease'.

With virtually no risk to the patient of injury or death, and no risk to the practitioner of being sued for medical malpractice, you might have thought doctors would have appreciated the work and the repeat business. In fact, they loathed it. Therapeutic massage was exhausting and required skills that were difficult and usually time-consuming. Demand was huge. If you could go to your doctor complaining of hysteria and be treated with the gift of an orgasm, is there any woman in history who would not make this complaint?

By the turn of the 20th century, the vibrator went into mass-production and there were models powered by batteries and mains electricity. To keep up with the demand, some physicians built vibratory operating theatres, with women being treated simultaneously on 20 beds. This was a booming business.

What's the buzz? Tell me what's happening!

Within 15 years, manufacturers began marketing the vibrator as a home appliance. It was sold to women as a health and relaxation aid. In a 1918 catalogue, the giant American company Sears & Roebuck advertised it as an 'Aid that Every Woman Appreciates' or as ' A delightful companion'.

The fundamental issue was the absence of any understanding between women and men and the latter's fear of a woman's sexuality. Even the word 'oestrogen' comes from the Greek for 'frenzy', 'hysteria' and 'suffering in the womb'. Mistrust of a woman's sexuality has been going on for a very, very long time.

An education

We can thank William H. Masters and Virginia E. Johnson's *The Human Sexual Response* (1966) and *Human Sexual Inadequacy* (1970), Alex Comfort's *The Joy of Sex* (the first illustrated sex manual for the masses, published in 1972), and then Shere Hite's *The Hite Report* (1976) for providing the world with a degree in sex education. Luckily, this took place while the 'me' generation – was coming of age.

These books brought to our attention the fact that over 75 per cent of women did not reach orgasm through penetration, and highlighted the importance of the clitoris in sexual stimulation. In particular, *The Hite Report* dispelled the myth of vaginal orgasms once and for all. Men became educated that good lovers fell into two categories: incompetent and competent, the first being self-interested, the second being desirous of giving pleasure. Learning that there was a clitoris that needed to be stroked, licked, blown upon or tapped in order to arouse pleasure determined whether a man graduated with a First in how to satisfy a woman.

Making sex pleasurable again

Testosterone is the hormonal 'rocket fuel' that gives both men and women their sex drive. It also helps to maintain bone mass and create higher levels of energy and muscle strength. Rising testosterone in adolescent boys and girls marks the beginning of their sexual urge to have intercourse. Guys just have a lot more of it. In fact, men produce about 20 times more testosterone than women, which probably explains why men think about sex roughly 250 times more than we do each week. If you don't have any libido, you might want to talk to your doctor about embarking on some type of testosterone therapy, which will kick-start your sex drive. The negative side of this sort of treatment is that it can lead to increased breast cancer, facial hair, acne and weight gain. You might also find yourself wanting to be in bed all afternoon with your vibrator when you have a hundred other things on your 'to do' list!

By the time most women have gone through meno-pause, they will have lost up to 70 per cent of their testosterone. Around the same time, the men in their life could have lost up to 60 per cent of theirs. However, even at these new diminished levels, male interest in sex will still be dramatically higher than ours.

I want to share the story of one woman who at the age of 54 had fallen in love again and was about to remarry. She was nervous about her new relationship because she loved her soon-to-be husband so much, but had completely lost her sex drive when she went through menopause. She went to her doctor, who prescribed a testosterone cream to rub into the skin on the inside of her arm. She had heard from a friend that if she rubbed it directly onto her clitoris she would fire up her dormant libido. Her clitoris grew literally to the size of a plum and it took over two years for it to return to its normal size. The good news is that the effects did eventually wear off and she is still happily married. She was also prescribed the *correct* low-strength testosterone cream that could be applied directly to her clitoris with good results!

The medicalisation of sex

Even when we were first sexually active and orgasms were much easier to achieve, we still needed the moon to be in the

Seventh House and have Jupiter aligned with Mars for it to 'feel right'. Sex is not a mechanical process for most of us, which is why orgasm and libido are not well understood by the medical profession. Although doctors are testing new drugs to increase female libido and satisfaction, it is becoming increasingly evident that our sex drive is more complex and cannot simply be switched on.

Furthermore, according to Irwin Nazareth of University College Medical School, London, 40 per cent of 1000 women surveyed reported a lack or loss of sexual desire, but only a quarter regarded it as a problem. It is unlikely that men would have the same response to a diminishing sex drive. As one newly divorced 65-year-old woman said: 'For a man to admit that they are less interested in sex is saying, in malespeak, that he is no longer as virile as he once was. If 65-year-old men wanted to date 65-year-old women instead of women half their age, both men and women could be true to themselves.'

Sex is more mechanical for men. Perhaps this is the reason why it has been easier to invent cures for their sexual problems. When a man can't have an orgasm, it becomes a first-rate medical crisis and the whole drug industry spends billions to research and work out a cure.

With the invention of Viagra, there was an even greater medicalisation of sex. The big pharmaceutical companies want us to believe that they have a magic pill to allow us to maintain a strong sex drive for all eternity. When Viagra was introduced, it became the fastest-selling drug of all time. Why, then, is the rate of repeat prescriptions so low? Is there really a need for this drug or are the increased expectations of our sexualised, 'stay-young' culture driving men to seek help? Is medical intervention the happy ending we are supposed to be dreaming about?

Sex and the post-menopausal woman

In all of this, I think it is important to think of yourself once again as a pioneer. In the early 20th century the average life expectancy for women was 49 and most women did not live long enough to go through menopause. Sex during post-menopause, then, is a relatively new phenomenon. We are also the first generation of women to go through menopause and benefit from the sexual revolution.

Our mothers, aunts and grandmothers never talked about sex in a way that was relevant to our lives today. Just about the time our mothers were going through 'the change', we, their daughters, were starting to discover our own sexuality. They might have thought it wasn't a good idea to discuss what they viewed as the end of their sexual life when ours were just beginning. Of course, it was just as likely that sex was a taboo subject and simply not discussed. The end result is that we have had to work out the problems of post-menopause for ourselves. Having at least one or two mentors who are 10 or 20 years older will help. If your mother is still alive, try to have a conversation with her about this.

Is penetrative sex mandatory for a long, healthy and happy marriage or any close relationship? Or are intimacy and sensuality the most important elements of a loving relationship? The bestselling *Sex Tips for Straight Women from a Gay Man*, by Dan Anderson and Maggie Berman, provides techniques and advice for women on how to drive a man crazy in bed without penetrative sex. It is amusing, educational and worth reading. We all know how sexually charged a great make-out session is, or to have our breasts gently touched or our necks stroked. Is there a woman alive who has ever said 'no' to oral sex?

Women do not need penetrative sex to have intimacy, but we do need intimacy. The mental and physical health benefits are huge. Although biology and culture incline women towards male/female intimacy to begin with, once the 'breeding season' is over all bets are off. It has become evident to me in the process of writing this book that many women in their 40s, 50s and 60s leave their husbands and find love again with a woman.

Human beings were created to love and protect each other, and we all need companionship. The fact is that we are all living longer. This means that we have to continue to change, adapt and redefine our sexual needs for more years than we originally bargained for.

My top 10 tips

1. Talk to your husband/partner about any sexual difficulties you might have. He might surprise you by coming up with a brilliant solution. If sex has been painful for a while, you might have an emotional and mental block about it, even if you love your partner and want to make love. Talking can open up other possibilities, and help to remove the block.

2. Experiment with different positions that might not cause as much discomfort. Some sexual positions allow you to control the depth of penetration.

3. Prior to bed, take a warm bath together, using relaxing bath oils. Some oils, such as rose, have been shown to increase sexual feelings and libido in both men and women and also to balance hormones and increase vaginal secretions during sex.

4. Try a vaginal lubricant or natural vitamin E capsules to help with vaginal dryness. It could make all the difference. If this doesn't work, ask your doctor about some of the other options – either traditional HRT or localised treatments, such as oestrogen creams, pessaries containing bio-identical hormones, or a vaginal ring.

5. Remember to encourage lots of foreplay. For many, this can be better than sex. Oral sex is at the top of any wish list!

6. Buy a vibrator. Just do it and thank me later. Every woman can climax and have multiple orgasms at *any* age if the circumstances are right. You might get the urge when your husband is not around, so make sure you have plenty of

quiet time to figure out what excites you. Then show your partner what you really like. Most women who go out and buy a vibrator find having an orgasm is much easier. If you don't want to go to a sex shop and be waited on in their back room, you can order via the internet.

7. The more toys the better. See how excited your partner gets at the mention of them. If he isn't the kind of man who usually likes to talk, broach this subject and you'll enjoy a conversation that lasts for hours. You will definitely feel better when you have talked more. Take the stress out of Christmas and Hanukkah and start writing a wishlist of what you both *really* desire. This will be a lot better than the toaster and blender he bought for you last year, and the socks and cologne you chose for him.

8. If you have no sex drive, talk to your doctor about the possibility of using testosterone cream or other possible pharmaceutical choices. There might be other issues affecting your sex drive, such as the quality of your relationship, how you feel about your body, and the amount of stress in your life.

9. Remember to do your Kegel exercises (see page 32). They provide the best workout to strengthen your pelvic floor muscles, which help support the uterus, bladder and bowel. They also help to keep the lining of your vagina in shape.

10. Do not run away from your problems. The elephant in the room is only going to get bigger, and it might not just be about what is going on with *your* hormones: your partner might be experiencing a drop in his testosterone levels too. This means fewer sperm, erections that take longer to achieve and are less hard than they used to be, a decreased ejaculation force, and a lower sex drive. Be prepared for the day he has the desire but not the ability. He will certainly be completely freaked out and worried about his manhood. Treat him as you would like to be treated.

About 30 years ago the comedienne Gilda Radner did a skit about premature ejaculation on the show *Saturday Night Live*. I have never forgotten it. She was dressed like Dr Ruth and looked at the camera and asked, 'What do you say to your husband when he prematurely ejaculates? (a) Shall we try again? or (b) Was it good for you? or (c) You selfish pork face! I will never be satisfied!' The answer was, of course, c.

When we were younger we could laugh at jokes about sexual dysfunction, but in reality we now need to be encouraging and sympathetic. For ways of supporting your andropausal, as in male menopausal, partner, see the next chapter.

CHAPTER NINE

Rediscovering love with your andropausal man

'A long marriage is two people trying to dance a duet and two solos at the same time.'

Anne Taylor Fleming, Marriage: A Duet

Whether you still have children living at home, or your last child has finally flown the nest, you could be looking at the man with whom you are sharing breakfast and realise that you don't know him very well. In the process of raising children, pursuing a career, keeping up with friends and the everyday hustle and bustle of life, you might not only have lost a connection with yourself, but also with your partner. Is it possible to rediscover why you fell in love and married in the first place?

If you have lost the spark or have simply forgotten what it is about him that excites you, you will need to spend some time finding new common ground and ways to reconnect again. Of course, if this were easy, the statistics would be different. At present, 40 per cent of all divorces take place over the age of 50, with 60 per cent of them initiated by women.

There were a few challenging years for both of you, as your body and mind went through the change. The stress, bad moods, floating anxiety and what appeared to him to be a schizophrenic personality are finally behind you. Let's face it – if *you* felt that you were living on an emotional roller-coaster, *he* experienced it too. This was part of the everyday reality of living with you.

If you are in a relationship where there is mutual respect and trust, and he hasn't left yet, he is not going anywhere. However, he might not want to spend time with his irrational, bad-tempered partner. The man in your life might even have grown to fear you, as he won't be sure which person will be greeting him at any given time – the caring, fun-loving and steadfast woman he married, or the ill-tempered, complaining and irritable person he has come to know in the past few years.

He learned how to tolerate your moods and make the best of the situation. But now you're more stable, *you* are not sure. You have begun to wonder what life would be like without him. Is your mind playing tricks on you or do you really feel this way? Does going through menopause, having your children leave the nest, and rediscovering purpose outside the home mean your relationship also has to change?

At this point in time you should be having the time of your life together. Why do so many marriages break up just about now, when you finally have your great pal back for the first time since your kids were born?

A hundred years ago, early death meant that marriage was for life. Women did not live long enough to decide they didn't have the life they wanted or to see their husbands run off with a younger model. Today women have more choices, more independence, more freedom and the opportunity to have more fun than ever before. Perhaps the brain transformation that takes place after menopause, propelling women forward to establish new relationships and create new passions, is nature's way of looking after older women.

Women do not simply wake up one morning after 20 or 25 years of marriage, look at their husbands and say, 'I want out. I want a divorce.' This usually occurs after years of being in an unhappy, unequal marriage. For some, it feels as if they are waking up out of a haze. They realise that going solo will ultimately be better than living with an unappreciative, self-centred bore for the rest of their life.

Some may be luckier. At about the same time that you are hitting your post-menopausal stride, the man who was too busy to remember to phone home is now looking at you to be his hang-out friend. You are now the person with whom he wants to cook, walk the dog, exercise and have lunch. Having spent your adult life caring for others and sublimating your own personal time and interest for the good of the whole family, you are now confronted with a husband who wants to be with you. Ironically, this all coincides with your new urge to explore the world beyond your home, and to rediscover things about yourself that have been dormant for years.

This is undoubtedly one of the greatest challenges that a long-term relationship or marriage faces during these years. If you are married to a decent and kind man and just need to put a spark back into your marriage, don't make the mistake that so many men and women do and devalue the relationship you have been dedicated and committed to for the past 20 or 30 years.

Does male menopause really exist?

Perhaps we should be asking ourselves what our husband or partner is experiencing at this point in his life. What you might not realise is that he may be going through his own kind of menopause. I don't mean mid-life crisis – I mean male menopause, which is also called 'andropause' or 'hypogonadism'. Male menopause occurs when the testosterone levels begin to drop; this can create many of the same symptoms that women experience during menopause.

According to a study entitled 'Male Andropause: Myth, Reality and Treatment' in the *International Journal of Sexual Medicine*, the typical symptoms of andropause are:

- Decreased erectile capacity (if your husband doesn't wake up with an early morning erection, chances are he is suffering from a testosterone deficiency).

- Diminished sexual desire.

- Decrease in intellectual activity.

- Fatigue.

- Depression.

- Decrease in lean body mass.

- Skin alterations.

- Decrease in body hair.

- Decrease in bone mineral density that results in osteoporosis.

- Increase in visceral fat and obesity.

According to a study released by the University of Sheffield Medical School, testosterone starts a slow but steady decline in a man around his 40th birthday. Other studies indicate that around one in three men suffers from andropause. Unlike female menopause, though, andropause rarely causes men to lose their fertility. Testosterone will continue to be produced, as will sperm, giving a man the ability to father children well into his 80s.

This is not the whole story. A 2007 study conducted by the University of California San Diego School of Medicine found that men with low levels of testosterone are more likely to die prematurely from all causes. 'The trouble with testosterone is that everyone just thinks it's a sex hormone,' says Hugh Jones, Professor of Andrology at the University of Sheffield, 'but it actually affects other organs too.' Research shows that boosting testosterone can improve the body's ability to control diseases, improve mood and increase muscle mass.

There is more and more research to support the belief that significant numbers of men do experience a decline in hormones in their middle and later years. But don't rush out to buy the man in your life testosterone supplements. If you give a man testosterone, the body converts it to oestrogen, one of the primary causes of an enlarged prostate. Just as it took almost a half a century to analyse and understand the effects of hormone replacement therapies on women, the same will be true in the discovery of testosterone replacement therapy (TRT) for men. In the meantime, research indicates that testosterone levels tend to be higher in men who exercise regularly and significantly lower in men who are couch potatoes.

A brief history of andropause

Doctors long suspected that a man's virility would be affected by the removal of his testicles, but this was not confirmed until 1849, when a German professor, Dr Arnold Berthold, did several experiments involving castration and testes replacement in roosters. He also discovered that the effects of losing the testes could be reversed by implanting another rooster's testicles into the cavity of the one he castrated. Berthold's work was the beginning of the study of hormones.

Coming up with medical solutions to restore male virility has been an ongoing challenge for the medical community. From the 1880s to the 1920s, physicians from Paris to Vienna to New York took to grafting the testes of monkeys onto ageing men in the hope of restoring youth and efficiency. Isolating the testosterone hormone was much more difficult. It took until 1935, when the German biochemist Adolf Butenandt isolated the testosterone molecule in his laboratory. He received the Nobel Prize for his discovery. His work led to the development of synthetic testosterone products, known as 'anabolic steroids'. Yes, the same ones that bodybuilders and misguided athletes use to pack on muscle and build strength to win gold and silver metals, and which subsequently cover them in shame when traces are discovered in their bloodstream.

The first study on male andropause, by two American doctors – Carl Heller and Gordon Meyers – was published in the *Journal of the American Medical Association* in 1944. It reported the effectiveness of testosterone treatment in helping what they described as the male symptoms of female menopause, but no one took it seriously. Men were unwilling to accept that they could go through male menopause, so the research was swept under the carpet.

Jed Diamond, author of *Male Menopause* and *Surviving Male Menopause,* says andropause 'can wreak havoc on ageing men'. He maintains that men suffering from it are usually diagnosed with something else, such as depression, and prescribed an antidepressant, when in fact this type of medication will only exacerbate the problem.

Is the man in your life going through andropause?

To work out whether your husband or partner is suffering from the symptoms of andropause, ask yourself these questions:

- Does he have a decreased sex drive?
- Is he lacking energy?
- Does he have reduced strength or endurance?
- Has he lost his zest for life?
- Is he constantly questioning his values, accomplishments and the direction of his life?
- Is he unusually grumpy?
- Are his erections less strong?
- Has his ability to play sports deteriorated?
- Is he falling asleep after dinner?

If you have answered yes to at least five of these questions, chances are the man in your life is suffering from andropause and might benefit from testosterone therapy.

Just mention the possibility of male menopause at a dinner party and you will see men either puffing themselves out, smirking at the ridiculousness of the thought, or squirming in their seats, desperate to talk about something else. Men, in general, do not want to believe that their testosterone supplies could start to dwindle. They would rather leave menopause to the female gender. I think one of the reasons that men like to date younger women is that it gives them a false sense of their own virility, which is not necessarily in sync with their own dwindling testosterone level.

Another reason for the 'sugar daddy' phenomenon could be that men who don't have diminishing testosterone levels have a stronger sex drive than the women they have been with for the past 20 or 30 years. To find a woman whose sex drive matches their own, they need a much younger model. Of course, he is wearing pyjamas and reading his book at 10 p.m. while she has her dancing shoes on and is heading for the clubs.

Every man has a feminine side

Although gender is predetermined at the moment of conception, it is believed that all foetuses are female for the first six weeks after conception. If a baby is going to be male, the appropriate genitals form at this point.

Taking this one step further, if all males start as females and, as they grow older, begin to lose the 'essence' (testosterone) that makes them male, they once again become closer to being female. In fact, by the time a man is 60, he will have more oestrogen in his body than you will in yours!

Similarly, as women lose their oestrogen and progesterone (the hormones that make them female), it makes them more like males. After all those years of feeling we are totally and mind-bogglingly different from the man with whom we share our life, we may finally be more alike than at any other time. Could the last 30 or 40 years of our life be the time when both men and women have more in common than ever before?

Is this the time when we can finally make peace with the male brain?

On this basis, it makes sense that we should try to stay together and rediscover the best in each other and ourselves. Being together and operating as a team as you journey through some exciting but challenging later years could be the best investment you have ever made.

If you are looking across the table at your partner and wondering who he is, recall your shared history: the sleepless nights, career changes, health scares, financial ups and downs, school entrance exams, deaths, new lives and everything in between. Of course relationships change – and love changes too – but do you really want to unlove someone at this point in your life?

What's love got to do with it?

Love, as we well know, is one of life's greatest mysteries. How can a rational person be attracted to a complete stranger, have sex with them the same night and end up walking down the aisle six months later? Alchemy, chemistry or serendipity? Luck has so much to do with how you and your husband grow old together. Why and how you fell in love will probably have nothing to do with the person to whom you are currently married.

My point is that if true love is largely irrational, do you want to throw away everything you have created with one man for someone else who could be equally annoying and complicated? When the writer Samuel Johnson heard about a man marrying for a second time after a very unhappy first marriage, he said, 'Second marriages are a triumph of hope over experience.' I know too many women who are thrice divorced because of the powerful, inexplicable intoxication called 'love'.

My favourite description of love appears in Louis de Bernières' book *Captain Corelli's Mandolin*:

❝ Love is a temporary madness. It erupts like an earthquake and then subsides. And when it subsides you have to make a decision. You have to work out whether your roots have become so entwined together that it is inconceivable that you should ever part. Because this is what love is ... Love itself is what is left over when being in love has burned away ... we had roots that grew towards each other underground, and when all the pretty blossom had fallen from our branches we found that we were one tree and not two. ❞

Louis de Bernières, Captain Corelli's Mandolin

Sharing our new world

Going through menopause helped many of us transform the way we look at the world and ourselves. We began focusing on our innate strengths and finally summoned the courage to stand up for ourselves and claim an equal footing with our partner. We became less interested in catering to everybody else's needs. This meant new rules and new boundaries for everybody. It is never too late to rewrite the rule book, as long as the rules are clear and fair.

This is not about narcissism or self-absorption, but rather about creating a new understanding. You spent much of the last 20 or 25 years giving your full attention to the day-to-day, microscopic needs of your immediate family. Of course you still love your children and husband, but cultivating your own passions and having a purpose will play a much bigger part in defining who you are, now and forever. This is the time when together you can focus on doing, not just being. It will give you both a wonderful opportunity to experience love in a new way – the love of each other and how it relates to the parts of your lives that you actively care about.

Over the past few years, it is likely that you used more of your free time to work out what would make you happier. Now, perhaps, he isn't working as hard; maybe he is semi- or completely retired, or he's lost his job in the latest round of redundancies. If he left his working career on his own terms, with his ego intact and adequate money, you are a lucky woman. He should be able, in time, to work out how to create a fulfilling life for himself and you. If he was pushed into a semi-retirement or asked to leave under a cloud, this process will be a lot more difficult. You will be dealing with a very bruised ego and a man not ready or sure how to make the most of his post-working life.

Of course, he has to be ready and open to share his life with you, and you need to be willing to share some of your life with him. There will be a period of decompression after he stops working, which will probably fall into the 'not fun and rather challenging' category. Make sure he knows you believe in his talents and are supportive of him.

If you are able to share with your partner some of what you have learned over the past few years, you'll be well on the road to rediscovering your best friend.

Whoever said you can't teach an old dog new tricks is just plain wrong. You are not teaching your partner how to reinvent himself – nor should you. Men hate it when their partners try to change them. This is not about changing him, it is about finding new ways to develop interests you will share together. In fact, it's not the 'learning of new tricks' that is the tricky part – it is the practice and incorporation of them into your life. You will both have to make an effort.

Begin to include him in the activities that *you* love. For example, take him to cookery lessons and cook with him in the evenings rather than you taking over the kitchen; take him to a Pilates or a spin class (he might end up really loving it); sign up for ballroom dancing or swing lessons; become a friend to a theatre or museum and see all of their shows and exhibitions; learn how to play bridge together; take golf or tennis lessons and set a regular date to play against each other or with another couple; sign up for a series of concerts or museum lectures. Initially, it doesn't matter what you do, as long as you include him in your life and make it fun.

Change for the better

Your relationship may be changing. For the past 10 years your husband may have been out playing football twice a week, rock climbing one night, cycling on another, and meeting up with his university friends once or twice a month. Maybe you both have separate interests that keep you active and stimulated, but not *together*.

How can you negotiate new boundaries with him so that he is happy and you are even happier? Are there ways to start having quality time together and function more as a unit on more nights of the week? Well, in a word, yes. What about asking him out on a date? Choose a night and book dinner and cinema tickets. Mark his diary in red so that he can't book anything else. If you agree to catch up and spend time together once every 10 days, you will create a new habit and something to which you both look forward.

You might need to be thick-skinned for a while as he works out how he wants to live the second half of his life. He senses you have changed and that a shift in the balance of your marriage has taken place. Your evolving equilibrium has little to do with him. Perhaps you are working in a new business venture, or have renegotiated your existing contract and are working hours that better suit you. All of this has given you more time to see your girlfriends, play tennis again, exercise regularly, slip off to see an art exhibition, spend some one-on-one time with your children, or engage in some charity work that makes you feel part of a bigger community. You have, at long last, your own agenda and are putting your needs first.

For better, for worse ... but not for lunch

I have heard many women say, 'I didn't marry him to have lunch with him every day!' Well, I understand that too, but if you can share the same philosophy about how to stay healthy and share a desire to find activities that give you both pleasure, it will help rekindle the spark. This is the easy stuff. Eating, exercise, finding hobbies that are fun and exciting, and sharing all this with your spouse is really very simple. Sharing life creates the ultimate bond and provides the basis for happiness.

What is difficult is how you react as a couple when disaster hits. You get sick. He gets sick. You lose a daughter or a son in a freak accident or to illness. Your lifetime savings get lost in the stock market or end up disappearing in a Ponzi scheme. Your best friend has a stroke and you need to be there for her and her family. Your or his elderly parents need much more attention. How you behave in challenging and tough times will be your making or your undoing. My husband has always said that the only way to judge someone's character is to see how they act under stress. When everything is going well, it is effortless to be generous, open-hearted, kind, compassionate and thoughtful.

If you have been functioning well, and you share the same core values and beliefs, you should be able to get through whatever adversity may strike. Providing emotional support, respecting each other's opinion and tolerating your differences, attempting to solve the problem by coming up with proactive solutions, and finding the courage and strength to help each other will ultimately make you closer.

Parallel worlds need to collide

When life is easy and you are happily cruising through each day, you may not even pause to consider that you have to make an effort. Maybe you have never actually thought about how to create opportunities for spending time together. Perhaps life worked well enough and you were both happy enough without making it a feature of your 'to-do' list. There was no need to make a fuss; he was not going anywhere and neither were you. Now, though, you need to make a conscious effort to ensure that your lives are lived together, not in parallel.

New beginnings

The years of desperately wanting your husband to start expressing his feelings really don't feature any more. You are equal partners now. He is no longer 'king of the castle' and you are your own person. What we want now is to take care of ourselves, live in the moment, be present, be happy with what we have, develop a purpose and a passion, rediscover the best in ourselves, stay connected to family and friends, and ensure that we are happy to spend some time alone each day. Friendship, forgiveness of each other's faults, shared values, support, loyalty and a sense of humour are the things that will make your proverbial empty house feel full again.

The choices facing women today are probably the most complex of any time in history. Women are deciding to get married later, and many don't think they need a man in the way they once did. Yet I do think the dream of living happily ever after lives on in a relationship where our talents are recognised, appreciated and valued by our partners.

Coming through to the other side of menopause and staying together will be deeply satisfying to you, your family and friends. You now have opportunities that could not have been imagined 50 years ago. The constantly changing landscape of the nuclear family means that your role as wife or companion will continue to be one of rediscovery and evolution. The payoff is priceless: a companion, a lover, a best friend, a husband to be with and explore the life you have been waiting to live.

My top 10 tips

1. Share your hopes and dreams for the future. Discuss where you want to live for the rest of your life, places you would like to travel to, the importance of doing things for yourself and each other and moving forward. The period of creating and growing your family while balancing your work life has shifted into a new phase – recapturing your dreams together.

2. Treat your other half as you would your closest friends, with respect and tolerance. The small things you do for each other end up making a big difference.

3. Never say 'never'. Ever.

4. Argue with respect and keep communicating by sharing your thoughts and showing him affection. Men like to be romanced too!

5. Choose your battles carefully. Some fights are worth fighting because they can solve problems. Otherwise, just live with it; you will both be happier.

6. Make time for the two of you and make sure you do things you both enjoy. Exercising together is time well spent – you are doing something great for yourselves and for each other.

7. Relationships are not easy. Dishonesty breeds distrust, which can kill a marriage. Keep lines of communication open, and if you have a problem, make sure you communicate clearly so your partner understands what is bothering you. Men have never been very good at reading women's minds.

8. Trust does not appear overnight, but it can disappear overnight. Trust is one of the most important parts of any good relationship. If it is lost, it can take a long time to create

it again. If you do something that could permanently create a lack of trust, be aware of the consequences.

9. Take time for yourself. It is important for both of you. Make sure you make time to cultivate your passion and have a purpose that gives meaning to you. You can give more to a relationship when you give more to yourself.

10. Nobody is perfect and both of you are going to make mistakes. However, there may come a time when you cannot forgive any more. There has been too much damage for too long and you are ready to re-evaluate your marriage. Take it slowly. You might find in time that you can forgive not only him, but yourself as well, by establishing new ground rules for the rest of your lives.

We change and then change again in the second half of life. Hopefully, you will have married a man with whom you share the same core values and beliefs so that you can find each other again. Those values will include your views on what makes a loving relationship – the importance of family, honesty, compassion, empathy, fidelity – and your views on money, drinking and drugs and your definition of trust and respect.

If you have a clash of values, there has probably been trouble brewing between you for a long time. When serious life issues are staring you in the face, it may just crack the relationship wide open, leading you towards a collision and then a break-up. Professional help will definitely be needed in the form of therapy and/or rehabilitation to try to repair the damage. You might come to the conclusion that separation and possibly divorce are your only solutions. For more about that, see Chapter 11.

CHAPTER TEN

New rules of dating for the post-menopausal single woman

'When dating someone, are there rules? You bet there are. These dating rules apply to every relationship, no matter if it's new or long-term, casual or serious.'

Ellen Fein and Sherrie Schneider,
The Complete Book of Rules

D id your mother ever tell you that the secret to getting a boy to fall in love with you was to smile a lot, look fascinated by whatever he said, and earnestly nod your head in agreement whenever he gave his opinions? Did she also say that if you did all of this, the man of your dreams would fall truly, madly, deeply in love with you, sweep you off your feet and in just a matter of months you would be walking down the aisle in your beautiful white wedding dress, saying your vows and be his princess for evermore? Did she by any chance mention that Cinderella resides in your home town and lived happily ever after?

What your mother should have told you is if you think being 'helpful', nice' and 'understanding' is the way to a man's heart and mutual love, think again. Dating and keeping a man interested and attentive is a bit like sport – make sure you play fair, but play to win. How can you make this happen? By setting the ground rules early. My advice is to avoid being too acquiescent and compliant, stand up for yourself, let people know what you stand for, and take just the right amount of crap – not too much and not too little.

If you adopt this attitude, it will help reverse the downward cycle of most failed relationships, where you do everything in your power to keep him interested (using all your strategies to please him), but it doesn't make the connection any closer to the man you have 'fallen in love' with. Then anger, resentment and frustration follow. You blame yourself, and decide the solution is to work even harder. But the relationship keeps getting worse.

Most men actually love strong women. If asked, they will say they would like a bright but compliant woman. But don't listen to what they say, watch the successful marriages and relationships around you. Men who are allowed to walk all over their submissive partners will do just that. The threat of a relationship going pear-shaped is never far away.

If you are in a new relationship (one that began in the past year), and it started off with you doing all the smiling, giggling and nodding, then you may need to ask yourself – are you getting what you need and at what cost? If you are not, tell him. If he engages in a long conversation, you can start to think that this relationship will last for a while.

Now is the time to establish a solid foundation based on your unique qualities – your passion and purpose, your sense of humour, your kindness, your character and who you really are. This part of your life is about change and liberation. What could be more liberating than being loved for who you are?

Grim fairy tales

Fairy tales can come true, but only with a good dose of reality thrown in. There are some harsh truths you will need to take on board to ensure you make things happen the way you want them to.

Is the fairy tale 'The Gingerbread Man' about a boy inside a man who can't make a commitment? 'Run, run, as fast as you can. You can't catch me, I'm the gingerbread man.'

Rule 1: Men only truly value a woman they have to work hard to get

It doesn't matter if you are newly divorced, newly widowed or have never been married, the rule stays the same: a man only truly values a woman when he has to work hard to get her attention and affection. Why? Because he really does not want to lose you once he has worked so hard to catch you. He perceives you as independent and strong and wants to have you by his side. You are now the woman of his dreams.

A little tough love in the beginning will go a long way in his desire to nurture and keep you happy. If a relationship is founded on this premise, you will be able to love him with an intensity that will not make him feel suffocated or overwhelmed because he will love you back with equal passion.

WHAT IS YOUR HISTORY WITH MEN?

Did you always hope to get married but never quite made it down the aisle? After every blind date do you promise yourself it will be different, yet find yourself in the same place after a few weeks – he stops calling and you don't have a date on Saturday night?

Or are you recently divorced? Did you divorce your husband because you got bored? Did you fall out of love because he wasn't dynamic enough for you? Or did he meet someone else? Was he a constant philanderer and you finally had enough?

Or are you a widow? Do you have wonderful and loving memories of your husband? Was he your best friend and companion? Or did you never *really* know him?

If you believe finding true love exists only in fairy tales, keep reading. This chapter is about making the man of your dreams love you the way you always dreamt of being loved. Why do some women have their girlfriends, husband or boyfriend saying yes to anything and everything they ask for, even to requests you might think unreasonable? Why do some of your friends have their phones ringing off the hook with invitations to openings, drinks parties and weekends away and others are always doing the calling and reaching out?

Is there a way you can be interesting and attractive to both men and women? It is important to act and look smart, but you certainly do not need a PhD to do this. Girlfriends, this is not about being book smart. This is about life smart – how to start a conversation and keep it interesting. Both men and women eventually feel suffocated by needy partners, and this will kill most relationships. The key to being in a good, loving long-term relationship is being independent, having interests and passions that you share together, and ones you do apart.

THE POISON APPLE

No man wants to be with a desperate woman. He can feel it. In fact the whole room can feel it. Recently, I was at a party with very interesting people floating around. I was there with a girlfriend who has always been single and still believes in the fairy tale ending. When we walked in there was this incredibly attractive guy who stared at her as she moved around the room. I told her, 'He is staring at you and is seriously attractive.' She said, 'I'm going to go to the bar and casually say hello to him.' I said, 'Stay here with me and make him come to you.' At that moment he walked over and introduced himself to us.

'Hi, my name is Tom. I'm feeling a little uncomfortable right now. This party is like a who's who of successful bankers. I *was* a vice president in private wealth management at Morgan Stanley, but lost my job during the last round of layoffs. I'm sort of in between jobs.'

Now there are a million and one things she could have said after that, but without skipping a beat, my friend said, 'Well, as long as we're playing True Confessions, I'm a scriptwriter – but in between relationships. I have never been married but I am really okay with it and really, really happy'. If she had meant what she said, it would have been fine. It was the neediness vibe that made Mr Tall Dark and Handsome and currently unemployed excuse himself after about five minutes and run for the hills.

Rule 2: Never call a man to ask him out on a date

Ultimately, no man will value you if you are too available or you are doing the asking. He must call you. Don't think for a second it will be okay if you call him. It goes with Rule 1, but as you can see, it is different. Never accept a date in the afternoon for that evening, or even for two days away. You are busy. The cooler, more detached and self-contained you are in the beginning, the more intriguing you will be to him. Don't rush to call him back when he phones. Remember, you are very busy. You have a life that you are very happy to fit him into when you can! And please, use your best manners when you apologise that you didn't have time to call him back when he phones again to see if you are free on Friday night.

In the beginning – the first month or so – you must always treat the man you are dating as someone you like but aren't terribly interested in. Flirt, joke, entertain him with your sense of humour, but make sure you keep gently pushing him away. Be kind, be interested (without the nodding head, please!), but in no way turn on the motor and start revving your engine. Please do not hold onto his every word. Set your own agenda. Make sure he knows what your interests are and make sure he bends over backwards to cater to what you like to do.

You can never initiate a call to him in the first month of dating him. Only after you are in a relationship, one that is truly and firmly established, can you start to let your guard down a little. If you have to, call him, it should be to discuss some complication about seeing him, such as you are double-booked but you do want to see him. Could you meet slightly later because you have somewhere to go to first? This qualifies as a phone call that you could initiate.

Make him value you by having the best time with him when you are together, but saying goodbye gracefully at the end of the evening. This isn't a game, but a strategy to ensure that he will value you later on in the relationship (if *you* want it to go that far). More importantly, this will also give you more time to figure out if he is really a man of substance or just someone with whom you are infatuated.

Rule 3: Make sure he is doing most of the running and is happy to do so

You may wonder why so many demanding women end up getting their man and keeping him. I think you need to consider what it means to be 'demanding'. If you are happy in your relationship and from the beginning were unavailable at a moment's notice to see him, encouraged him to do most of the running, all the asking and all the calling, he will continue to want to make you happy throughout your courtship. High maintenance is in the eyes of the beholder. If and when he loves you, he will love everything about you and want to please you. If you are the person he truly values, the tickets to the play you casually mentioned will probably appear under your pillow. You won't be considered high maintenance. You will be the woman he wants to make happy by doing the 'little things'.

If a man is not romantic, not emotionally there, flirts with other women and does not pay compliments, this makes a woman insecure and can make her demanding because she isn't getting enough attention. I am *definitely* not talking about that kind of 'demanding'. If you find yourself in that sort of relationship, you need to think seriously about ending it or how to reset the boundaries. Splitting up and not taking his calls for a week or two could help. Dating other men is another good way to get his attention and make him rethink just how wonderful you are. Even then, if he really is just a good-looking, vacuous shit, you should dump him and move on.

Most men love high-maintenance sports cars, even if driving over a bump too quickly means that the engine drops out. It doesn't matter; the love of that car takes over all rational thinking. This is going to be you … You are his Maserati, Ferrari, Jaguar or Aston Martin DB9.

Rule 4: Make sure it feels right

A friend of mine recently said, 'There is a difference between wanting a man in your bed and wanting him forever.' I thought this was a clever thing to say, but it did not ring true. Because we were the baby boomers, born between 1946 and 1964, we grew up watching *Coronation Street* and *The Dick van Dyke Show* and observing the morality they portrayed. Consequently, there is still part of our subconscious telling us that sex should be meaningful.

Can you remember back when you were a teenager and your mother discussed sex and dating with you? I remember my mother saying to me, 'Why would anyone buy the cow if they can get the milk for free?'

Now fast-forward 35 or 40 years. Any man who doesn't respect your wishes to take intimacy at a pace you feel comfortable with and says any variation on 'You are being ridiculous! Don't you want just to have some fun?' – run a mile. Any man who says you are too old to be acting like a virgin should make your skin crawl, just as it did when your 17-year-old boyfriend begged you to have sex, claiming that if you didn't, you would give him blue balls.

If he is just looking to get laid – and even if you are too – is this the kind of guy you want to share your bed with, even for a moment? Sex for the sake of sex simply doesn't feel right or good. If you think he is just good for dinner and a shag, and you are 100 per cent clear about this, then *carpe diem* and go for it. Otherwise, this sort of primeval encounter might make you feel less than you are. No man should ever make you feel like used goods.

THE MAGIC KISS

In my 20s and 30s, when I used to date, I always found kissing to be the most exciting and important act of intimacy. After a couple of dates, if I liked his sense of humour and the kissing felt right, somehow the rest would fall into place. If the kiss didn't ignite a passion or make my heart go pitter-patter, there was really no need to carry on dating. I don't believe this changes at 50, 60, 70 or 90 years of age. Please remember to value yourself, and don't change your own beliefs just because some man wants you to. Do what feels right for you. Just because you are a post-menopausal woman, it doesn't mean you should change the morals you have always felt comfortable with. The code of ethics and your beliefs have been with you your whole life. You must listen to your heart *and* your mind as they will be what ultimately guides you.

Rule 5: For the first few dates, make sure he is the one paying

Call me old-fashioned, but no matter how much money you have, when a man asks you out (remember, *you* will not be doing the asking), he should pay. A date is a date. If you end up having a fantastic time on your first date and he asks you out again, don't think about pulling out your purse. Not on a first, second or third date. If it is within his means and he is not prepared to pay for supper or a movie, to be quite frank, he couldn't possibly have a clue how to look after you emotionally. I do not care how charming, charismatic or gorgeous he might be: he and whatever else you might be fantasising about is a complete non-starter.

If you have a great job and he doesn't, then, after a month or so, of course you must pay your share and treat him from time to time. The key to how the relationship will develop in the longer term is in the first months. He has to show he values you not only by asking you out on dates, but by organising great nights out that you will enjoy. Enough said.

Rule 6: If you're feeling jealous, do not show it

Okay girls, this is a big one. If he makes you feel jealous by going away with his male friends three weekends in a row or flirting with an attractive woman or a friend of yours at a cocktail party, you are absolutely justified to feel this way. However, you cannot whine, even if you are feeling needy and when you talk about your feelings, your voice should sound unemotional, like 'I am going downstairs to make myself a cup of tea'. He should not know that you are upset or angry. He should just know that his behaviour isn't what you want in a relationship, and if this is how he chooses to behave, he really should find someone else.

There is nothing as attractive to a man as a woman who doesn't need him. If, after having this little chat, he doesn't alter his behaviour at all, go and have fun with your friends or go out on a date with the man you met at your cooking class. You must never start nitpicking, nagging and complaining because you are jealous. Men hate women who whine. Show him you don't need him and the odds are overwhelmingly in your favour that he will stop this behaviour.

Rule 7: Keep yourself a challenge

Men think they want compliant women but end up marrying or staying with women who challenge them. Men are hunters, remember? If they get anything too easily, they become bored and ultimately move on. A man will date a sexy and dutiful woman for a few months, but will ultimately lose interest. This can happen after marriage, but the writing is on the wall.

Men can and do get confused that 'nice' means 'weak'. Most men will take advantage of your sweet nature and ultimately move on to greener pastures. Make sure you know how to stand up for yourself. Don't ever be afraid to voice your opinions, and when you say 'no', mean 'no'.

Most interesting men are attracted to strong, independent and feisty women. Even if you are all those things, making yourself too available takes away the challenge. You will be taking away what a man has been programmed to do for thousands of years – hunt and chase. Sure, put out the olive branch, but don't call, write or send him flowers; it has to be him chasing you.

Rule 8: Less is more

Don't talk too much. Dating is not a chance to practise dictating your memoirs. He doesn't need to know about your past blunders. He definitely does not need to know that you think you weigh a few kilos more than you should, or that your best bedtime friend over the past two years has been your vibrator.

Less is more. Never reveal information about yourself that you don't have to. Be interesting and have something interesting to talk about. Talk about something besides yourself: a new book you have read, a debate, a talk or a lecture you just went to about politics, the media or the arts, or a discussion you heard on Radio 4. Have an opinion about what is happening in the world, quote something from *The Week* magazine, talk about a new play that just opened at your local theatre, or a new exhibition you've just seen at the Victoria & Albert Museum.

Always maintain a dignified silence when it comes to ex-husbands or past relationships. Speak with integrity. Don't ever speak badly against yourself or your ex, and don't confide in a man you are just getting to know. Your tales of woe are actually quite boring. Nobody except your mother and your closest girlfriend is really interested. Don't talk about people, unless it is about his children and yours. Even then, there is plenty of opportunity to do this when you actually get to know each other a lot better.

Rule 9: Keep a close eye on the balance of power

Never be obviously controlling, and don't ever embarrass or undermine him in public. He will feel emasculated and will grow to resent you.

Your strength must come from within; otherwise, you will look like some pushy woman who is always trying to get her way and control every situation. Strong does not mean pushy. Strong means strength of character, always trying your best, having well-informed opinions, and communicating clearly so you can avoid misunderstandings and drama. Taking the high road and galvanising your inner strength will give you control of your life to help you celebrate not only yourself, but each other. Make an effort to function as a team. If each thinks they are giving over 50 per cent, this will ultimately be a recipe for a wonderful partnership.

Rule 10: Trust, like and respect

The cleverest man I ever worked for in business told me that you can't be in a successful relationship (or be a successful leader) unless you have at least two of three stool legs standing firm. These legs are trust, like (not 'love'?) and respect.

If you want a lasting and deep relationship, it is best if you can tick all three of these boxes. So think about it. Do you, after dating him for a couple of months, think you can trust him? Do you respect him? And, do you actually like him? If you can't answer yes to at least two, if not all three, questions, it's not a relationship worth investing any more time or emotional energy in.

Make sure you share the same core values and beliefs. It is fine that you have opposite personalities because they can complement each other. However, if there is a clash of core values, the relationship is a disaster waiting to happen.

Advice between friends

When I asked my Kitchen Round Table group what they believed to be the basis of a good relationship, they came up with several more recommendations that don't really qualify as rules, but more like sensible advice you would share with your best friends.

- Think back to what was important to you when you were younger and try to date that kind of person again. If what you value most is a sense of humour, a sense of curiosity, or being with someone whose ego allows them to get a kick out of what you are trying to achieve, don't lose sight of what is important. You must feel a spark, that surge of electricity for who he is, not for his big cheque book or how successful he is in business. Don't try to stick a square peg in a round hole. If it isn't right, it never will be. You want to be with a man who says, 'If she is happy, I am too.'

- Even if you can remember the past, you may be condemned to repeat it. No matter how old you are, you are not immune to making bad choices. Falling in love can happen at any age, and you might think that now you are older, more stable, wiser and confident, you will bring new things to your latest relationship – that this time it will be different. You could be right, but be aware. You have probably been attracted to the same kind of man your whole life and use the same routine to promote intimacy. Try to put your old tricks away and start afresh with a determination to do things differently.

- Never take a guy seriously if his best friend also tried to date you. Even if he is persistent and acts desperate to be with you, nine times out of 10 he is usually out to prove something to his friend. You are the prize, but not necessarily the one he values for the right reasons.

- Watch out when a man says at the end of a first date that he is looking to remarry. Pinch yourself hard and remind yourself that every man in the world believes mentioning marriage to a 50+ woman is her greatest aphrodisiac. It is like offering candy to a baby. Don't fall for it. You know the mark of a successful relationship is not its outcome but the process and the quality of the relationship.

- Never ask a man if you can meet his children. Believe me, he will think of it when the time is right and he is good and ready.

- Never introduce a man to your children if you are even the tiniest bit unsure about him or the relationship. Your kids will sense the fear and offer up some major reasons as to why this guy is not right for you. If your children really dislike the man you are dating, do give it some serious thought.

- Even though you can't get pregnant, practise safe sex by making him wear a condom. You must protect yourself against sexually transmitted diseases (STDs) during menopause and post-menopause. Use a latex condom *every* time you have sex. You may be surprised to discover just how many partners he has had in his adult life.

- Never move in with him – ever. Only join households after you are married.

- If a guy doesn't drive you home or wait for you to get safely indoors, don't bother going out with him again.

- Don't date a married man. Truly, at this point in the game, life *really* is too short.

- Never say anything you might regret. Hurtful words are remembered a lot longer than kind words. Don't use sarcasm to make a point. Speak with integrity and say only what you want to say. Remember, he really cannot read your mind, so subtle hints are pointless and can easily be misinterpreted.

- Never mention anything to do with getting married again, looking for a diamond ring or anything else around this theme unless he has brought it up and there is a mutual commitment and understanding.

- Don't ever pretend to be anything more than you are. You are enough!

- Nobody can ever complete you, but a man should certainly complement who you are, your interests and personality. Just make sure you put yourself in places where you might meet Mr. Right. Keep an open mind. Mr. Right will more than likely not be what you were expecting him to be.

- Don't change who you are for anyone. If he doesn't appreciate your sense of humour, get a kick out of your sense of fun, listen to your opinions and be willing to discuss them, as you would with a best friend, the relationship is never going to work. Look elsewhere.

Where is the fairest one of all?

Before you can even think about applying the rules and advice above to your life, you have to be open and put yourself in a position where you could meet someone you might want to date. Many women find the process of dating again daunting, particularly if they are newly widowed or recently divorced. Remember you are not going to be every man's cup of tea but you will be someone's. If you find the whole process of meeting new men difficult, there are other ways than going to speed-dating dinners or being set up by your well-meaning friends.

Remember, get out of the house. Take public transport, walk a friend's dog, even become a volunteer for a prostate cancer charity! Anything that puts you in the company of interesting men. Don't rule out internet dating or even using a dating agency, where you can anonymously pick and choose from potential candidates who share your interests. Please make safety your greatest priority: ensure a friend or family member knows where you are and that you meet your date in a restaurant or some other public place. Internet dating is an explosive business but beware – everyone on the internet is tall, dark, handsome, interesting and successful.

Fairy tale with a modern twist?

Cinderella had to battle her awful stepmother and stepsisters to find her prince. Your obstacles may be when too much liquor, loneliness, passion and infatuation take over and you jump into bed with a man you hardly know but think is great. Is there a magical genie willing to grant you one wish?

Depending how you handle yourself moving forward, the magic can happen again. If he does call again (remember, *you* are not doing the calling), you will have to sound very happy to hear from him, but you are unavailable on the night he asks you out. If he likes you, he will call again and then you can say yes, as long as it is not for that evening or the following evening. When you see him for a second time, make sure he is doing most of the running. You will need to figure out if he is someone you actually want to sleep with. Note: That will definitely not happen on this date!

If you are reading this and saying to yourself, 'This is just wrong. It is all so dishonest. Why do I have to hold back? Why can't it just be mutual? Why do I have to fight my impulses, my desire to see him, call him, talk to him the way I would like to? Why do I need to play this ridiculous game? It is so wrong.' My advice is to try it. You might be surprised by the results.

You may find some of my ideas old-fashioned, but the truth is that we *are* old-fashioned. These are the values our mothers raised us with. Although the world has shifted quite a bit in the mores of dating, our moral compass has been pointing north for a long time. By incorporating the above guidelines into your new dating life and living your 'new five-a-day', you will be giving yourself the best chance to be in a loving, mutually respectful and fulfilling relationship and, quite possibly, live happily ever after.

CHAPTER ELEVEN

Preparing for separation and divorce

'Divorce is like an amputation: you survive it, but there is less of you.'

Margaret Atwood, author

Your children have grown up. They have either left home or act as if they are ready to leave home, and you finally have more time. You are ready to rediscover life with the man you have been married to for the past 20-something years. Perhaps take the trips you always dreamt of together; take tennis or bridge lessons together, maybe even have lunch together every once in a while?

Here is the reality check. In the UK 43 per cent of marriages end in divorce and over 50 per cent of divorces occur after the age of 45. Please take a moment to imagine what divorce would mean for you and how you would live out the rest of your life. If you haven't been paying attention and you think the spark has gone, now is as good a time as any to think about how to re-energise your relationship. If *you* think something is missing, it is likely that he thinks so too.

If he does, what is he thinking and doing about it? Well, one in 10 men you know right now will be interviewing divorce lawyers and thinking about getting (if he hasn't already) a newer version of the woman he is currently married to: a feisty, energetic, non-complaining woman (the one you used to be) about half his age plus 10 years. Do the maths. You will find the age of the newer model of you.

Divorce statistics prove that the overall rate of divorce is falling for the first time since 1981, but between 1997 and 2007 divorce in England and Wales in the 45-plus age group rose by more than 30 per cent. And that latter figure is set to rise still further in the decade ahead, as women feel less inclined to put up with relationships in which they are unhappy.

According to a nationwide study commissioned by the American Association of Retired Persons (AARP), women in their 40s, 50s and 60s initiate over 60 per cent of all divorces. Just as surprising, one quarter of the husbands involved were completely shocked – they never saw it coming. The fact of the matter is that women in their middle years often begin to visualise what life would look like if they were on their own.

Although women generally initiate more divorces than men, this is not something they do enthusiastically. It is more that they have come to the end of their patience with things that they have put up with for too long. 'I am not going to put up with his philandering, drinking and lack of consideration the rest of my life.' 'I need someone who at least acts like they want to be with me.' 'We *really* don't have anything in common. I'm not sure we ever did.' 'We stopped liking each other long ago.' 'He is controlling to the point of abusive.' 'He is constantly criticising me.' These are just some of reasons why women ultimately file for divorce.

When the vows of marriage were first written, the promise to 'love and to cherish till death us do part' generally meant you bound yourself to a spouse for 15 or 20 years because the chances were that one of you would be dead by the ripe old age of 35, through disease, hard physical labour or childbirth. Today life expectancy is on the rise and Professor Sarah Harper, Director of the Oxford Institute of Ageing, believes that before too long we will be living well into our 90s. This means when we now say 'I do', we are talking about spending six decades together!

The media, psychologists, philosophers, Church and society have for centuries tried to brainwash us with the idea of the perfect marriage – and for each generation it changes. We waste hours on end fantasising about what the perfect marriage should and could be. Should we be having sex twice a week, twice a month or twice a year? Where sex is concerned, when it doesn't live up to the expectations we've been fed, we fantasise about other people's marriages and relationships and how much better their sex life is than our own.

> How can the institution of marriage survive? Is there a difference between married love and romantic love that works for both men and women? Is it grounds for divorce if you would rather watch the finals of *The X Factor* than have sex?

Another problem in the marriage sweepstakes is the different ways in which men and women cope with their issues. Women like to talk things out, while most men resist these upfront emotional discussions. We know when we stop talking that we have given up. This should be a big warning sign for men. Of course, men leave for some of the same reasons. When asked, they will say they wanted out because they were tired of being 'nagged to death', 'micromanaged in the home' and 'got at the whole time'. They also say they want more regular sex. They want a new mating partner.

More than likely, the seeds of destruction and discontent were starting to take root in your 30s, and by your early 40s they were sprouting. By the time your children start leaving home, the sprouts will have grown into weeds that are strangling and destroying your marriage. You are a bit like Little Red Riding Hood lost in the forest, where the big bad wolf of a different name, the divorce court, will be waiting to devour you.

Why and how does a marriage go wrong?

I have a few theories about how a well thought-out decision can turn into a big mistake:

Mistake 1: The dynamic wife morphs into a doormat

Some men like to marry their intellectual equals and then somehow convince their vivacious, talented and accomplished new wife that what they really want is a woman who will sublimate, for the love of their new expanding family, everything she has worked for and accomplished during the first 30 or 35 years of her life. As he rewrote the rules early on, she morphed into something she never thought possible – something more akin to a Stepford Wife than a Female Eunuch. He became more dictatorial about his demands. He wanted time at the weekend to play golf, or generally more time to himself. He wanted supper ready when he got home, a dinner party organised for his boss at a moment's notice, and the children to have perfect table manners. If they didn't, it was your fault.

The woman he married – the self-motivated, bright, determined, bubbly, vibrant woman – ended up defining herself through their children and her husband's successes and failures, and with this came a loss of identity. The dream of building an equal partnership and becoming the person she always thought she would vanished into thin air.

For the record, choosing to be a stay-at-home mum and deciding not to work does not in any way equate to losing your own life and turning into a Stepford Wife. However, if you let yourself be marginalised, there will be trouble brewing in paradise before too long. If you live vicariously through your children and husband and don't have anything to call your own, small problems will become big problems.

Some women, when they decide to stop working, become obsessed with the minutiae of their children's lives because their children become their whole life. Trust me, your husband does not want to spend his evenings discussing what qualifies as a healthy school lunch, how you engineered a whole new social life for yourself by finessing a friendship for your daughter with the new Apple Paltrow Martin of her class, or how you found a music coach so little James could have a singing part in his Year 3 play. It just gets dull after a while.

Anyone can all fill a day with 'busy', but how good does that make you feel? If you aren't filling your day with something purposeful for yourself while your husband goes from strength to strength and continues moving up the career ladder, he could wake up one day and not recognise the passive, subservient woman he is married to. His female colleagues and clients remind him of the person you used to be. He may begin to lose respect for you and think there is a lot more to life than the doormat he now has for a wife. He will start to look elsewhere.

Mistake 2: The doormat rebels

This is the flip side of mistake number 1. Your husband has put you in the role of *hausfrau* and house manager. You are suffering from extreme boredom. Your husband is working all hours and you feel neglected and unloved. You have too much time on your hands and excitement is lurking just around the corner. Someone catches your eye at the supermarket, the gym, at a party – anywhere. He really isn't at all suitable, but he ignites a flame in you that has all but gone out. You are ready to throw away everything you have created for the past 20-plus years just to remember what it feels like not to be his shadow, his servant, his cook, his chief washer-up, the person who is always there for him. You start having an affair to know what it's like to feel alive again. By the time he realises he created this situation, you are at the point of no return. And to add insult to injury, he ends up making your life hell because he blames you for the breakdown of the marriage.

Mistake 3: The trophy becomes tarnished

There are actually men who get married because they can't believe that you, this incredible woman, could be in love with them. By marrying this 'trophy', his friends and colleagues will think, 'That lucky bastard. How did he even get her to look at him twice?' She is a reflection of his macho, successful and powerful side. Anybody this superficial really doesn't care about making you happy in the long run. He wanted a woman he could manipulate and dominate. If this is you, it might have worked well for a while, but as the years kept coming, the beautiful, young and nubile trophy transformed into an insecure, middle-aged woman. You lost whatever value you had for him. Your very existence has started to annoy him because you are no longer the arm candy that validates him to his world. You evolved into his personal assistant – there to fulfil his every wish. He doesn't respect you. He now wants to replace you with another beautiful young woman to make him feel youthful and virile.

Mistake 4: You didn't think ahead

You got married because it was always your dream to have the diamond ring, the white wedding and children. Your biological clock was ticking but you really didn't think it through. You thought about the wedding but not the marriage that followed. Or you married too young, hoping it would work out. Maybe you married for lust, and when it faded you realised you didn't really have much in common with the man you married. You never stopped to think, 'When everything else is stripped away, do I like him?' You realised soon after you said 'I do' that you didn't really share the same values, interests or life goals. You stopped respecting him long ago. You simply married for the wrong reason.

Mistake 5: You develop attention deficit disorder

You married for the right reasons. You shared some great times. You shared common values and interests. Everyone thought you were a good couple. You raised your children together. The last one has just left home. You take a deep breath of self-satisfaction. You have a good husband, wonderful kids, everyone has their health, you have an interesting and eclectic group of friends and interests outside the home. You are content.

You did not always give him the attention he would have liked. Intimacy and sex slipped lower and lower down your list of priorities. You were too busy juggling the kids, job, friends and school/charity work. You really put the brakes on sex when you started to go through menopause, but he seemed pretty good-natured about it. It was a trade-off for his ever-increasing travel schedule and work demands that kept him at the office late into the night.

Then one day you find the hotel and restaurant receipts, the credit card statement showing a purchase from Agent Provocateur, dozens of extremely personal emails and a long trail of deceit. Does he love her? Can you forgive him? Is this something you both are willing and able to fix?

Mistake 6: The breadwinner is living on emotional crumbs

What was simply a job became a career. You were like a duck to water, discovering that you actually liked working and were good at it. After five years you couldn't afford to give up work as you were the major breadwinner in the family. Although you never flaunted it, he felt marginalised and emasculated. He became unhappy and so did you. You had a couple of affairs that made you feel even more miserable. You grew apart. You knew the marriage was over. He never appreciated the sacrifices you made for him and the family. It was clear that life would be easier to make a go of without him.

Working full time can help to keep the balance in a relationship but certainly adds its own stresses and marital strains. Long before you go through menopause, working and managing a family feels exhausting and makes sex seem more of a chore than a pleasure. All you want is a lie-in. When the dishwasher breaks down unexpectedly (washing machines and dishwashers never stop working during business hours), getting it repaired can send even the most organised woman into psychiatric care.

For women who work full time, most of our non-working day is still spent organising the children. Whether you want to acknowledge it publicly or not, 90 per cent of the childcare duties rest firmly in your domain. Daily tasks used to range from organising day-care, booking tumble tots sessions, ensuring school uniforms fit and are labelled to arranging music, ballet or football lessons. As the children grew up, you chauffeured them at 7 a.m. on a Saturday morning to sport fixtures or other school activities, organised special shopping afternoons, helped with the PTA, booked them tables at clubs, and kitted out college rooms and flats at IKEA.

You overcompensated for everything. It was like walking a tightrope. The stress and strains of having too much on your plate and the inequalities of your pay cheques took the marriage to breaking point.

> 6 We choose a partner who helps us to grow and sometimes we reach a point where the relationship has run its course and no more growth is possible. 9
>
> *Penny Mallison, Kitchen Round Table member*

You need more reasons?

There are other reasons why you might want to leave a marriage. Sometimes we can't agree on children and how to raise them. Sometimes there are problems with the in-laws, other family members or friends that can lead to the big D. Of course, there can be a conflict of personal beliefs and philosophy that you are no longer willing to tolerate. Financial issues, such as how money should be spent, not having enough, not speaking openly about finances, keeping money in his and her accounts, or using money as a way to control a marriage, can become more significant.

All of these scenarios will have severe consequences unless the problems are addressed quickly and you start remembering together why you first fell in love and rediscover the passions that made life exciting for you as a couple and as individuals.

Even when the problems seem overwhelming, it does not necessarily lead to divorce. Can you rewrite some of the rules so they work for both of you? Hopes of reconciliation will rise and fall, come and go. If you think your relationship can be rebalanced, both you and your husband need to sit down and figure out new boundaries. To rediscover the best in each other takes commitment and focus. It's not going to get any better unless you both want to make it better. It might feel like an easier solution to drift apart than to make the effort to glue it back together.

When you can't remember why you have stayed married for the past 25 years, because you look at him and think he's boring, stupid and certainly not king of the castle any more, slow down. Take a deep breath. Is he a good person? Is he kind? Could you renew your commitment to each other by finding a marriage counsellor to help you understand that you are each 50 per cent of the problem? Could you try to remember why you fell in love with him in the first place and attempt to put differences aside?

The million-pound question is how to keep the embers burning bright. If you have mutual respect, trust and truly like each other, chances are – unless Rachel Weisz walked into his office half-naked and asked to have his babies – you two will share a very long and happy life together.

What *was* important changes

What has been important to women in their late 20s, 30s and 40s – keeping the family together, keeping the peace and keeping the children safe – is replaced by embracing new challenges and putting their own needs and desires before the family's. As women move through and out of the haze of menopause, a simplicity, a clearness, a sense of purpose and a balanced perspective of what is important take over. The 'self' part becomes much more important in the second half of your life: self-love, self-respect and self-worth. Can the hormonal changes in the menopausal brain be blamed for the seismic shift?

Recently, in one week alone, I heard about four couples who decided to separate. The women were between the ages of 48 and 62. Three of the four couples no longer had children living at home. In two of the four cases, the divorce was initiated by the wife. Some women, especially those in higher-income couples, feel pushed to petition for the split, to take back control after a husband announces he is leaving her for someone else. As one woman said to me, 'I am so getting in there first!'

Of course, being married is not everything; in fact, it is nothing if you are in a horrible marriage. If you are in a truly bad marriage, I am all for throwing in the towel. A woman who has tolerated living with a serial philanderer, an abusive alcoholic, or a completely self-centred husband for the good of the family will simply put the brakes on. A post-menopausal woman might well be prepared to go through the hassle of divorce and the difficulty of readjusting to living alone rather than live the rest of her life being made to feel less than she thinks she is. Her husband may be thinking that this is just another phase, but she knows differently. This is a forever state of mind!

You now want a husband who is a friend and partner in every sense of the word; otherwise, living alone starts sounding like a better and better choice. Acting like the family housekeeper is no longer part of your remit. He needs to share in these responsibilities. This is what a good partnership is all about. Although some of your relationship may only require tweaking, some could involve a serious rewriting of the rules.

If only it were as easy as 1-2-3

When it comes to a marriage breaking down, the reasons fall into three basic categories.

1. You and your husband drift apart and possibly into extra-marital affairs through lack of common interests, different personal beliefs or philosophies, feeling neglected, lack of passion or sex, or financial issues.

2. Your marriage involves physical or emotional abuse. Some of this could be the reason for extra-marital affairs, but a woman who is in physical danger from her spouse should not stay with him.

3. Your marriage involves drug and/or alcohol abuse (this affects men and women equally). Alcoholics or drug addicts know that the bottle or their substance of choice will always come first, well ahead of their partner and the family. Addicts always promise change, but unless they make a commitment and agree to a programme of rehabilitation, there is little chance of a marriage surviving.

Point number one also includes another reason that has attracted increasing attention over the past few years. Some firmly avowed heterosexual men and women discover same-sex attraction, and this completely changes their lives and their marriages. One only has to look at the success of the 2010 movie *The Kids Are All Right* to understand that same-sex love has gone mainstream. Several men and women I spoke with did not identify themselves as gay; they simply found love with someone of their own sex. For many women, it is more about the person they meet than embracing their gay identity. Many high-profile women, from *Sex in the City* actress Cynthia Nixon to retailer Mary Portas, have spoken publicly about finding happiness, deep connections and uncomplicated sex with another woman.

When change means changing your relationship

If you decide you do want change and don't want to be part of your marriage any more, make sure you think through what it will be like living alone, having your children split their holidays between you and your soon-to-be ex, losing your built-in hang-out companion, having a lot less money, and possibly a long and expensive legal battle.

According to top divorce solicitor Catherine Bedford of the firm Lee & Thompson, 'Where it is the husband who has and controls all the finances, it is common for him to go into shock if it is the wife who wants a divorce, and he feels angry. However, at some point, a switch will flick and he will go into "business deal mode" and his aim will be to get the best price. To achieve this, he may well grind his wife down by delaying things, controlling the money and making her "earn" the divorce. This kind of man knows that his wife does not have the stomach to fight or the money to pay lawyers to fight for her unless she borrows from a bank and/or goes through lengthy, stressful court proceedings to get the money.' Be prepared.

Ultimately, divorce and the loss of a spouse are so much more painful than the process it takes to forgive someone. Is there any chance of reconciliation? Getting through the second half of your life with your life partner may be easier than going it alone. Do you really want to get divorced or is the discontent a cry to nurture the relationship and give it some much-needed attention? Do you still love him? Can a proper trial separation make both of you reconsider? You never imagined going through all those years to end up here. After laying it all out for him, you may be very vulnerable and he may be promising big changes. Please don't fall for it and don't go back until there is true evidence of change.

Simple rules for separation

Separation is a time for re-evaluation, to spend some time apart and take stock, to focus on yourself and your marriage. At the end of a predetermined period you will have a clearer idea of how you want to move forward. Separation is a time of emotional turmoil and you cannot be expected to act in a reasonable or sane manner until things settle down. You are more than likely feeling miserable, but so is he. A male friend said to me six months after his divorce, 'I was so lost in myself after divorce. I didn't know who I was any more. I was terrified. It was almost like a death of my hopes and dreams.'

Rules are difficult to follow when you are feeling vindictive, hurt, alone and nervous about your financial well-being. Whether you are the one initiating the separation or the one having it thrust upon you, please follow these 10 important rules.

1. See a professional marriage counsellor

It is too difficult for just the two of you to tackle all the problems you have both swept under the carpet for many years. Find a professional marriage counsellor or couples therapist who comes highly recommended: that step will be worth its weight in gold. A few counselling sessions are the least you owe a 20- or 30-year marriage. A good therapist can help both of you to look at things objectively and see what you need to focus on. The therapist will be there to mediate the hurt feelings and disappointments. Trying to defend your own corner is as productive as driving on a road to nowhere.

A woman told me that after years of tolerating her husband's unprovoked and unpredictable verbally abusive rages, she could not take it any more. He saw them as mere temper tantrums; she felt depleted and hurt by them. She finally drew the line in the sand and insisted they go to counselling together. What she took as a constructive measure to give their marriage a future, he perceived as an attack. His way of protecting himself from the 'attack of having to go to counselling' was to seek out other women to prove to himself that he was fine. Her husband's newly exposed lack of integrity finally gave her the strength to pull the plug on her volatile marriage. For her, the therapy worked, though not as she expected or hoped it would. The caveat here is to be aware of what therapy may unearth. It will not always have happy endings.

2. Always see a solicitor

If you don't see a solicitor, the other rules don't have as much value. This has to be a priority. There are many men out there who take advice about what their legal position is long (in some cases years) before a divorce. Then they sort their finances out accordingly.

A matrimonial solicitor told me the following extreme tale of woe. You won't cry for either of the parties involved, but it makes a point. A man stopped loving his wife. He knew he would divorce her one day, so he made preparations for this eventuality. When he sold his company for £20 million, he told her he sold it for £5 million. He put £5 million into an onshore bank account and £15 million into an offshore account. Then he divorced her two years later, and it was only after she hired a private detective that she found out the truth.

Before separating you should always find out where you stand legally. Always talk to a lawyer about what is on your mind because you may well find that some of the things you want to say to your husband would be to your disadvantage. Sometimes it is best not to put the other side on notice that there is a problem. It is imperative you are informed. Information is power.

Finally, don't use your solicitor as your therapist. You won't thank him or her for it when you get the bill. Your lawyer should advise you on the nuances of your legal rights, but is there to be someone with whom you feel comfortable.

3. Be brave

This is going to be one of the hardest things you will ever have to do. For most women, separation is completely outside their comfort zone. For the time being, the way forward is to fight fire with fire – in other words, appear to be as strong as your partner. He needs to relearn (if he has forgotten) to respect and value you. If you still love him and have any hopes of reconciliation, he needs to see you as strong, feisty and challenging. You need to show him you are not his passive security blanket and that you are very capable of living without him. Yes, of course you never imagined that you would go through all these years to end up here. After laying it all out for him, you may be feeling very vulnerable. Be strong!

4. Separate quickly

If you are the aggrieved party, ask him to move out early enough in the process to make him think long and hard about what he is losing before he has time to put all his ducks in a row. A man who loses his anchor quickly finds his way back to the safest dock – and that is you.

5. Don't sort-of separate

If you decide to separate, do it properly. Don't give him the pleasure of your company, your cooking, your warmth or anything he has grown used to as part of the marriage package. If he has a key to the family house, he should only use it in absolute emergencies and should respect your space as a distant acquaintance would.

One woman I interviewed who went through the whole process of separating, selling the family home and setting up two households could not cut the marriage 'umbilical cord'. After all of this, she would invite him every night of the week to join her and the children for supper, he would sit around and read the paper, not help with the dishes, and act like they were married. This 'separation' lasted for four years. He divorced her when it suited him – when his eldest son went off to university and he'd left his high-powered banking job and was earning a tenth of what he had been three years earlier. When she still had a chance of making him realise what life would be like without her, she wasn't brave enough to separate formally. In the end, she discovered her fear of being single was actually much worse than being single again.

6. Have a clear and mutual understanding about dating

This is a huge issue. Your husband might expect you to be completely faithful to the marriage during separation. Then again, his definition of dating may be different from yours. He may think that dating is synonymous with sex, while you may be thinking dinner and a movie. Once you have discussed the ground rules and have a clear understanding and mutual agreement, you must honour it. Please try to put yourself out there and go on a few dates. You might meet someone you enjoy being with, or you might realise that, with a few rules rewritten, the man you would like to spend the second half of your life with is the man you have been married to all along.

7. Do not have sex with your husband while you are separated.

This is especially true if you have had a wonderful sexual relationship. The idea is to spend time away from the marriage and each other. It really defeats the purpose of a trial separation if you sleep together. Make-up sex can be addictive, but remember that the issues that have created the breakdown of your marriage have not been resolved. Distance makes the heart grow fonder; making him want you and value you could be the key to a reconciliation.

8. Keep children out of your differences, always

Depending how old the children are, you might not have to decide which parent they live with and the role each of you will play in raising them. Nonetheless, children should be kept out of your differences during the trial separation and the divorce. It is confusing enough for them to figure out if you are together or apart. Living in limbo land is not something they like. You might not get along with their father, but it remains important for them to have the best relationship they can with him. They don't need to be involved with the nuances of your feelings or any issues and disagreements you are having.

9. Before a trial separation, see a solicitor about money

As one of you will be moving out, there will be additional expenditures, so there should be a clear understanding of who will use what money and for what purpose. If you don't trust your husband to provide support, or he fails to follow through, you will need to file for a legal separation. You should make an agreement that there will be no major purchases, no selling of marital assets and no large withdrawals of cash from joint accounts. Don't start think about mine and yours. There will be plenty of time for that. Maintain your dignity and self-respect.

10. Set a time limit for your trial separation

Try to think of this trial period as a good thing; a time to regroup, prioritise and discover a few self-truths. You will have to decide who will move out, where you or he will live and for how long. It should not be an open-ended separation After this pre-agreed period passes, either file for divorce, negotiate an extension of the trial period, or move back in together.

At the end of a separation, if you both think it makes sense, let the mistakes of the past be a learning experience. Studies have consistently shown that it is easier to grow old with someone who knows you well. You have already shared half a lifetime together. A friend, now in her 70s, said she ultimately couldn't get divorced because it gave her too much pleasure to have her grandchildren grow up visiting them together.

Will it be more painful to forgive each other or get divorced? A trial separation should give you a good opportunity to see the pros and cons of staying married. Hopefully, you both will have had enough time to reflect on mistakes made and have a chance to decide how to best move forward.

> 6 Pain nourishes courage. You can't be brave if you have only had wonderful things happen to you. 9 *Mary Tyler Moore, actress*

Let's say after going through this process that you really can't see a way forward together. You have thought about it and you actually feel more alone when he is at home sitting next to you than when he is away on a business trip. You are fighting constantly. You feel you are ready to move on with your life. You have actually grown to dislike him. You want to get divorced.

Before you leap ...

One last time, ask yourself the following questions:

- Do you actually need to get divorced?
- Can you solve your unhappiness in other ways?
- Could you be suffering from depression for medical reasons that pharmacology could solve?
- Is your view of your marriage and husband possibly being coloured by an imbalance in your hormones?
- Will the grass really be greener on the other side?
- Are there reasons to stay in the marriage?
- Could you sort out a different type of working relationship?

PREPARING FOR SEPARATION AND DIVORCE

If, after going through the process of a trial separation, you both come to a decision to end the marriage, your husband might decide to wage psychological warfare. This is particularly true if he is cuckolded, feels abandoned and thinks you have broken up the family. He might decide on dragging out the divorce proceedings just to hurt you. Remember, what doesn't kill you makes you stronger. Be prepared for any and all of the following:

- He might decide to turn the children against you by completely spoiling them – giving them things that you don't approve of or can't afford. That may mean serious clothes shopping, taking them to Paris or Venice for a special weekend, or out to supper at trendy restaurants. On the other hand, some men don't see their children much and forget they were fathers for the past 15 or 20 years of their lives.

- Your mutual friends might feel they need to take sides.

- He might promise to pay for something and then doesn't. He might agree to a plan and then cancel it at the last minute.

- He might decide to stop responding to your phone calls or emails.

- He might think it is appropriate to introduce your children to a woman he is casually dating and doesn't know well.

- He might do all the things and be everything you wanted him to be when you were married, just not with you.

- He might always say no to what you view as reasonable requests (such as switching weekends with you).

- He might end up dating a close friend of yours, or a close friend's sister.

- He might be very late in making payments. You will need money for expenses while you go through the divorce process, which can take on average two years. Your lawyer can arrange for an amount to be turned over to you to keep you solvent for a period of time.

- He might want you again when he realises how easy it has been for you to live without him. Think long and hard about that one. Remember, Elizabeth Taylor went back to Richard Burton and ending up divorcing him twice.

Divorce is about two things: money and the children

For starters, getting divorced is expensive. A top divorce lawyer currently charges £435 an hour. However much it cost you to get married, it will cost you at least three times that much to get divorced. If you end up going to trial, you will add another £30,000 to the total bill.

It is very important to find a good divorce lawyer, either by word of mouth or through *Chambers Directory of the Legal Profession*. Shop around and interview at least two or three. This will be the most important relationship you will be forming at the most difficult time of your life. Make sure when you choose your divorce lawyer that you select them on their ability and knowledge. They should have an excellent track record and be able to work hard on your behalf. A good divorce lawyer should be someone you trust and should understand what makes you tick.

Financial matters

Your lawyer will give you a Schedule of Expenditures form to figure out what you spend in a year on property, finances, household living, personal living expenses, car, leisure, children and other expenses. This will help you to work out how much money you will need to live on going forward, and how to spend less or save more if there is a shortfall when you and your spouse split up your joint assets and incomes. The legal divorce maintenance payments will take on average two years to sort out.

Listen to your solicitor. Jeremy Levison, senior partner in the family law firm Levison, Meltzer & Pigott, advises: 'Even if you are the one to fall out of love and initiate the divorce, don't give everything away out of guilt. Sooner, rather than later, your husband will still want his pound of flesh and try to take everything and more from you. Your soon-to-be ex-husband may try to brainwash you into believing that you will be left with nothing and that your children will be taken from you. The good news is that he cannot kick you out of the family home. The bad news is that you cannot kick him out either.'

Your divorce lawyer will also give you a Standard Financial form on which you need to give a clear disclosure of all your financial and other relevant circumstances. Do yourself a big favour; whatever financial documents have been kept at home, photocopy them and give them to a friend for safe-keeping. If you suspect your husband could be hiding money, prepare the necessary paperwork immediately to obtain protective orders and injunctions to stop him. If the house or other property is in his name, fill in land registry forms and protect your rights of occupation. If you don't trust your husband to do the right thing for you and the children, you should move all the money held in a joint account into your own name for emergency funds, and have your solicitor inform your husband.

Regarding the children

In 95 per cent of all cases, divorcing couples will come to a suitable and sensible arrangement about the children. In the other five per cent, women try using the children as weapons to inflict pain or revenge on the ex-husband. In a word, don't! As long as he is not unstable or dangerous, he should have access to the children and share in the responsibility for their lives.

However you got to this point in your lives together, be fair and understanding. This might be the hardest pill to swallow. All assets gained during the marriage should be equally shared, but allow your ex the dignity of keeping what he alone was responsible for acquiring before you ever came into the picture. You can't buy respect, so make sure you keep yours. At the end of all this, you will still have to deal with each other regarding the children and many other matters. Don't be less than who you really are. Life is long and you will have to live with yourself for a long time. Speak with integrity when asked about your ex. It doesn't make you look good to make him look bad.

Children repeat the mistakes of their parents because they learn what they live. Listed below are what I believe to be 10 fundamental truths to share with our daughters about falling in and out of love.

My top 10 tips

1. Marry for love, not for money or status. A friend of mine who manages a chain of upscale resorts and has seen it all says, 'When you marry for money you pay for it every day of your married life.'

2. Falling madly in love is dangerous. When you fall 'madly in like' you have a better chance of a successful and long marriage. You want your best friend by your side after the initial passion inevitably fades.

3. If you think you have found your love match, the sex is better than fantastic, and you are 100 per cent sure, take a deep breath and don't get married for at least six months. There is only one way this relationship can go and that is downhill. If, after six months, it is 80 per cent as good as when it started and you are still happy, start planning your wedding.

4. Be open to being set up by friends and family. A friend of mine and her three sisters were all introduced to their husbands by their mother.

5. Whether you get divorced or not, the chances are that more money will be needed as you get older, so work as many years as you can before and after you get married. Work until it becomes absolutely impossible for you to juggle growing children and a career. If you have a good career

before leaving work, your re-entry to the job market will be much easier.

6. Your chances of staying together improve dramatically if you marry someone whose parents haven't split up and were happily married. His role models were his parents, who worked out their differences and kept their marriage together.

7. Make sure you keep a bit of your own life while raising the children. Give yourself one night a week that is just for you: a trip to the gym, a book club, a dance or cooking class, or go to the movies, a concert or theatre with a girlfriend.

8. Never speak negatively about your husband, ex-husband or life partner in public. If you don't have something nice to say, keep your mouth shut.

9. Make sure you share the same core values. If you come to the relationship having different religious beliefs, make sure you discuss it and come to a mutually agreeable solution. If he is cheap and you are generous, you'd better talk about it sooner rather than later. Don't wait to have these conversations. You must overcome your fear of losing him and have the courage of your convictions. He must know early on that you will leave if certain things are not sorted out. Clarity early on will help to avoid bigger mistakes later.

10. If you decide to marry, you must figure out how to get along with his parents, family and best friends. If you realise this truth early, you won't have to suffer needlessly.

Getting divorced is like buying a home; it brings out the worst in people. Maintaining a dignified silence is the best way to help yourself and those affected to adjust to the split. Your children, other family members and close friends will need reassurance during the transition. How you support and help them may actually be the best predictor of your own future and how you heal wounds and move forward.

CHAPTER TWELVE

Facing up to loss

Putting the first half of your life behind you

'You gain strength, courage and confidence by every experience in which you really stop to look fear in the face. You are able to say to yourself, "I lived through this horror. I can take the next thing that comes along." You must do the thing you think you cannot do.'

Eleanor Roosevelt, US first lady

We know that people and things we love can disappear at any time. Loss, of course, comes in many forms: children leaving home; the end of fertility; health problems; lost youth and opportunities; dreams that no longer seem possible; the end of a marriage; the death of a parent, child, life partner or friend.

Loss can be defined as the end of the life you have always known, but also the beginning of a new and different life. Of course life will not be the same, but it will force you to redefine and rethink how to move forward with the rest of your life. This is where your new brain that heralded the onset of menopause kicks in. Of course loss is challenging, but this is the time to take a deep breath and start rediscovering your true passions and purpose. It will give your life direction, give you a sense of who you are and why you were put on this earth.

Loss is part of life. Loss is part of growth. It is also a time of rediscovery. Any loss will propel you to reassess who and what is important to you. Loss can free you to figure out what to do next.

Many of the women I interviewed said they were not afraid of their 50s or 60s, but became fearful in their 70s and 80s. Past fears, such as fear of flying, driving on the motorway, spiders, heights or public speaking, lessened or disappeared completely. But fear of how they would grow older became the primary fear, alongside a fear of not being able to fill the empty spaces when a loss happens.

However, when I asked women who had experienced recent loss about their fears, the response was fairly universal. 'The fear of the loss is much worse than the loss itself.' 'The loss forced me into action, so I was able to find a way to transcend the grief'. 'We are all stronger than we think we are.' 'We find courage that we don't know we have until we have to.'

A woman who was recently diagnosed with cancer and underwent a mastectomy explained why she elected not to have reconstructive surgery: 'I had been through a lot in the past year. Both my parents had died. I had a life-threatening episode of pneumonia the year before. When I was diagnosed with breast cancer and was told it could be solved by removing my breast, I thought, "Great. One potentially huge problem solved." I opted not to have reconstructive surgery. I figured my bosom fed my two daughters and had done its job.'

No matter what your loss is, the finality of it can make you feel as if you have lost everything for a while. But when the sadness lifts, you realise you have been given a new opportunity to reassess and make some choices that didn't seem available to you before. This is where your new five-a-day will help you to overcome the feelings that *everything* is lost.

Empty nest

The loss many women dread and that has no catastrophe attached to it is when our last child leaves home. I was going to devote a whole chapter to empty nest syndrome, but at first all I could come up with fitted into one paragraph:

> Your kids leave home. You cry for a week. You wake up and the gloom has lifted. A light bulb goes off in your brain. You have an epiphany. Your house stays clean and tidy. Dirty dishes don't get left on the sofa. Your best jacket is not rolled up in a ball at the back of your daughter's closet. You can go to dinner parties that start at 10.30 in the evening. You only need to go food shopping once a week. No one complains when there isn't any food in the refrigerator.

In the process of writing *The Second Half of Your Life*, I had regular gatherings with my Kitchen Round Table group to share ideas and information. They did not want me to belittle the realities of children leaving home and the physical loss of not having them there to love each day. The loss of being needed, having a purpose and knowing what the basic structure of each day will look like – the routine of dragging them out of bed, giving them breakfast, making their lunch, driving them to school, preparing dinner, helping with homework and nurturing and supporting them with each and every problem that arises. In a sense, this is a death of a life you lived. So I kept writing...

You now have more time to do whatever you want to do, and to explore things you have kept on hold for the past 20 plus years. Your children come back to visit and you think, 'Did we really raise these terrific people?' These nice, interesting adults are now happy to see you. Your children want to talk to you as much as you want to talk to them. They seem not only to have survived, but have somehow thrived during the 18 years they lived with you.

You realise they will always be your children. You still think about them, worry about them, and help whenever you can. They just don't live with you any more, and you hope they will start a nest of their own. Who they are now won't change, and acceptance becomes the rule of life. Your days of active parenting are over. You save your best book, *Helping Your Child Sleep through the Night* by Joanne Cuthbertson and Susan Schevill, for when they call you in desperation after three nights of being awakened every two hours by your beautiful new grandchild. A good empty-nesting parent never criticises or offers advice unless it has been asked for – especially if you want to see your children or grandchildren on days other than Christmas, Diwali or the first night of Hanukkah.

It dawns on you that you can finally do some of the things you always wanted to without the day-to-day restraints of having children, managing a busy household and holding down a job. A giddy sense of freedom may start to wash over you. You will mourn your loss every day, but this is replaced with an overwhelming urge to engage in dormant passions and hobbies. Your days of putting your eggs in everyone else's baskets are over. It is your time to balance the caring you do for others and the caring you do for yourself. This is your time to rediscover the best in yourself. You can now be a loving parent to yourself.

You don't have to have children to suffer from empty nest syndrome. It can also strike those whose home was once hyper-charged with activity but has now gone quiet, or when a routine that was second nature changes. Suddenly you are not sure what to do with yourself any more.

In the beginning, adjusting to your empty nest can feel like one step forward, two steps back. The separation for some is painful, for others just a dull throb. Preparing for this time and being consciously aware of what you need in your life will help you to identify how to cut the spiritual umbilical cord and acknowledge the need to move on. If you haven't prepared for it, you should start preparing now. Reread Chapter 1 and make your new five-a-day your life. You will need to start finding direction and a life focus. If you don't, you are going to be looking at premature ageing and a loss of everything you hold dear in your life.

Empty nest and empty marriage?

Empty nesters spend more time alone, so they have more time to micro-examine and analyse their lives. They will also spend more time with their husbands. This can either be wonderful for your relationship or bring to light how much you have grown apart. Problems that used to simmer just under the surface can start to bubble over. The timing of all this is horrible. Just as your children fly from the nest, the other most important relationship in your life, the one with your husband, starts to fall apart.

We all know there has been a huge increase in the number of divorces among couples married for 30 years or more. You might be attracted to the idea of reclaiming the TV remote control and not finding the toilet seat up in the middle of the night, but if you get divorced around the time your children leave home, your nest will be completely bare.

Now that you don't have any children to look after, don't fill the void by hyper-focusing on your husband. He may enjoy this for about a week, but it won't be good for you, him, or your relationship in the longer term. Find new activities you can do together and separately. If all else fails, get a pet. Dogs are always happy to see you when you get home. A pet can fill an emotional void and give you both a new shared activity.

Did you ever hear this joke?

Q: How can you tell who loves you more – your husband or your dog?

A: Put them both in the boot of your car for an hour. When you open it up, which one is really happy to see you?

The second half health challenge

In the first half of your life, you spend relatively little time thinking about your health. Then, in the second half, everything about your body seems to demand your attention: your bones, breasts, heart, blood pressure, skin, eyes and ears, teeth, the big 'C' – cancer, diabetes, cholesterol levels, fibroids, uterus, cervix and ovaries, sleep and memory. Study after study has shown that many of the health issues we view as typical of ageing can be slowed and even reversed by regular exercise and a diet of unprocessed foods.

If you haven't already started making these changes in your life, start now. While they're not a guarantee you won't contract these diseases, they will certainly decrease your chances. On the NHS Choices website (www.nhs.uk) it is estimated that almost 75 per cent, and in some cases 90 per cent, of cancers are related to how you live your life.

Cancer and menopause

As if all the hormonal changes that happen aren't enough to deal with, it seems as if every week someone we know is being diagnosed with cancer. Nobody wants to think about the possibility of getting cancer, but we are forced to. Almost 80 per cent of all cancers are diagnosed after the age of 50.

Although breast cancer is the most common cancer in women today, lung cancer is number two, followed by colorectal cancer (cancer of the colon and rectum). Other types of cancer also high on the list include cervical, endometrial, ovarian, bladder, vulval and vaginal. These are all affected by a woman's exposure to oestrogen and toxins, weight gain and lifestyle choices.

RISK FACTORS

When it comes to breast and other female cancers, there are some key risk factors that could make you more vulnerable:

- If you are over 50, but the risk doubles when you reach 65 years old.

- Family history of breast cancer in either a mother or sister.

- Taking hormone replacement therapy for more than five years.

- Early menstruation (before the age of 12) or late menopause (over the age of 55).

- Heavy alcohol consumption.

- Having breast cancer diagnosed in one breast increases the chances of developing cancer in the other breast.

A monthly self-check of your breasts should become as natural to you as brushing your teeth. You should know how your breasts normally feel and look. If you are not sure how to self-examine, please discuss this with your GP.

GENERAL HEALTH CHECK

A general health check-up every year is a must. Early detection of disease is the best way to deal with it. This is all about learning to take care of yourself. If you haven't had a general check-up for a while, call your GP now and book yourself an appointment. Tests should include:

- Blood pressure (for your heart health).

- Blood sugar (for diabetes).

- Faecal occult blood test (for colorectal health).

- Skin check, including the back of your legs, the soles of your feet and between your toes (for any moles or pigmented lesions of the skin).

When you see your gynaecologist for your yearly check-up, you should have a smear test and full pelvic and breast examinations. Depending on your medical history, you should have a mammogram every one or two years, and possibly an ultrasound. The latter can locate small, hard-to-find cancers that mammograms can't.

SURGICAL OPTIONS

Should breast cancer be detected, there are four surgical options available to you with regard to removing the cancer:

- **Lumpectomy** – the least invasive surgery to remove the tumour and a small amount of normal tissue around it.

- **Simple mastectomy** – removal of one or both breasts, breast tissue and nipple.

- **Modified radical mastectomy** – removal of the breast and the lymph nodes under the arm.

- **Radical mastectomy** – removal of the breast, lymph nodes and muscles behind the breast. This is no longer common and used only when there is no other treatment option available.

Today many women opt for reconstructive surgery, and many doctors perform this at the same time as the mastectomy. If and when the decision comes to remove a breast, this is where the mature menopausal brain kicks in. After being diagnosed with a rare form of breast cancer, a woman I interviewed said, 'I needed to take responsibility for my own breast cancer. It was only my breast that had cancer. I did not want it to spread to my marriage, my family and my friends. The loss of a breast did not create any negative feelings in me, which surprised me. It was inconsequential compared to the potential damage that could happen if I didn't keep my eye on the future and process the thoughts and emotions I had internally.'

Will there be a rainbow after the storm?

Most women I know like to control what they can. As our 'to do' list gets longer and our time compresses, we feel our lives spinning out of control. This causes our stress levels to rise. It also makes a serious dent in our sense of humour, ability to concentrate and our general outlook on life. Prolonged stress will rewire the brain, leaving you more vulnerable to anxiety and depression.

We all know what triggers our stress, and that can multiply tenfold when a serious disease is diagnosed. One woman who was recently diagnosed with lymphoma told me: 'When I found I was sick, my brain shut down. It was not equipped to hear about its own mortality. For a short while it feels like a death. The death of a life you once knew. But then you realise life must go on, and so shall I.'

Each person will process their illness differently. But it is a loss, and for however long you are undergoing treatment, there is a grieving. The process starts as shock, numbness, denial and disbelief. This is usually followed by some feeling of anger – why me? Then there is acknowledgement of the disease, a willingness to accept, a power to confront it, and finally a strength to cope with whatever it takes to get healthy and start living again. From the clouds a rainbow starts to appear.

A remarkable woman, Judy Dewinter, now chairwoman of Myeloma UK, was diagnosed with this rare type of cancer at the age of 33, and the treatment for it caused her to go through early menopause at the age of 34. On average, a typical myeloma patient has a life expectancy of three years after diagnosis. Judy's diagnosis was over 13 years ago. She said, 'After going into denial for a year, I knew the way I was going to get through this was by making my disease a purposeful and positive event. After a year my brain just kicked in. I had this overwhelming urge to figure out how to best use my skills and strengths to make a difference to other people with this disease. The new meaning I found was as a spokeswoman who could give value in terms of life and health. It kept me both sane and productive.'

In the second half of our life we sometimes worry that we have not made enough of a difference and didn't achieve our life's purpose. Finding purpose and passion and making it part of our everyday life gives strength, peace of mind and ultimately relief. It helps balance the spiritual, emotional and physical parts in each of us. It allows us to accept life for what it has been up until now and what it will be in the future. It helps remove the negative feelings of what you could or should have done.

This alone will not solve the regrets and sometimes bitterness that will keep your life from moving forward. You must also take care of yourself and make sure you exercise and eat primarily foods that come from the ground: fruits, vegetables and foods high in omega-3 fats (see page 112). Stay away from foods high in sugar, saturated fats and trans fats (see page 90). Do not overeat, and watch your intake of alcohol. You will increase your risk for virtually every disease known to womankind by being overweight or obese.

When someone you love gets sick

What if it isn't you that is sick, but someone important to you – your parents, your husband, your child, a life partner, a close friend? How can you help? Many women I interviewed said that even some of the people closest to them didn't know how to act or what to say when they first heard they were sick.

Being there for someone who is sick can help them reclaim some control, take the edge off their fear and give your relationship more importance in the future. The actor and director Orson Welles said, 'We're born alone, we live alone, we die alone. Only through our love and friendship can we create the illusion for the moment that we're not alone.' Although this may be true, the actress Kathy Bates said something much more profound in the movie *P.S. I Love You*. 'The thing to remember is if we are all alone, then we are all together in that too.'

What does this mean? It means taking the time to show love and friendship, to be physically there to lend a hand, or simply listen. Just sitting for a couple of hours can be a huge support. Writing a note is a lovely thing to do, but don't give open-ended offers of help, such as 'Call me if there's anything I can do'. Be proactive. Take food. Help with the laundry or other household chores. Drive your friend to medical appointments. Ask your husband to call your friend's husband and take him out to a movie or supper. Be present. Be positive when you can, but don't comment on things you know nothing about.

Many women have told me that friends, trying to be helpful, will say things such as, 'You are definitely going to beat this disease. I feel it in my bones. Really, stop worrying.' Although I think that sounds helpful and supportive, apparently it is incredibly annoying to someone who is sick. Their view is, 'What does she know? I don't want to hear her droning on about something she doesn't know anything about!' Far better to go online and find some helpful information so you can speak with greater knowledge and understanding.

My top 10 tips to help a sick friend

1. Be present. Be a good listener, but also a good talker. Bring positive news of your life and try not to be a burden by sharing depressing news.

2. Do not let a visit be something you tick off your 'to-do' list. Make it count and make it meaningful.

3. If someone close to you is going through chemotherapy and losing her hair, it's not only depressing for her, but is a

physical and outward announcement of being sick. If she doesn't have a good wig, do some research as to where she could get one, and take her to pick it out. Alternatively, take a gift of a beautiful scarf, a lovely candle, relaxing bath oils, new face cream or make-up. It can all help.

4. Talk to or email all your mutual friends and figure out a rota so that you all are updated on any health news. This gives everyone an opportunity to check in with each other. There was a fantastic rota created for a friend of mine who recently underwent chemotherapy. Friends would not only drive and accompany her to her chemotherapy sessions, but also knew which days of the month to take food and deliver meals.

5. Take a book and magazines you know your friend will enjoy reading after your visit.

6. Help tidy up the house.

7. Help with transportation. This can mean picking up children and other family members at the airport or railway station, or driving to and from the doctor's surgery.

8. Read poetry and play inspiring music. Download *Sand and Water*, *Look* and *Back to Love* by singer/songwriter Beth Neilsen Chapman. This will be a gift to your spirit whether you are healthy or sick.

9. Organise a girls' night in and rent a DVD. If you decide to watch *Terms of Endearment* or *The Notebook*, make sure you take a spare box of Kleenex. If it is your husband who is unwell, make certain you rent what he wants, which more than likely will be an old World War II film or one of *The Godfather* movies.

10. Be positive. Tell the people who are important to you that they are amazing and you love them. Nobody can hear that enough.

There is no time like the present. You do not need a cold blast of mortality to begin creating lasting legacies. But legacies don't happen overnight and they don't happen by accident. They are built over years of hard work and dedication, and can come in various forms. Financial legacies, for example, can support causes such as cancer research or a new building at your alma mater. Personal legacies can involve simply passing on the lessons you have learned to the people in your life.

It is never too late to spend time with the people you care about and to find new ways of communicating with them. Create a diary and begin writing down what you remember about growing up, your own parents, friends and boyfriends in secondary school and university, dreams and aspirations, and mistakes you made along the way. Maybe include why you fell in love and any tips on marriage you think could be helpful to the next generation later in life. Include special memories you have of your partner, children, family and friends.

Loss mirrors life. How we cope with our losses, no matter what they are, takes courage – the same courage we have drawn on to create the life we have made for ourselves thus far. I am not saying we should live every day as if it is our last because who has the energy to do that? Loss is as unpredictable as how we find our way back from it. It is how we re-emerge as a different person who has found the strength to heal, rediscover and find joy again that will determine how we live and appreciate all aspects of our life for the rest of our life.

CHAPTER THIRTEEN

Finance matters
Now more than ever

'Annual income twenty pounds, annual expenditure nineteen pounds nineteen and six, result happiness. Annual income twenty pounds, annual expenditure twenty pounds nought and six, result misery.'

Mr Micawber in David Copperfield *by Charles Dickens*

One way or another over the years you have learned something about money. Everyone's experience with money is different, but you won't find many people who will say money doesn't matter. The fact is that when you don't have enough money, it becomes more and more important.

Most married women leave the financial part of their lives to their husbands, with the exception of cheque writing, which usually falls under the woman's domain. This is because women believe their husbands are simply better than they are in the long term at financial planning and management, and think their family's interests will be better served this way. Because of this, many women do not have a clear idea about money and are ill equipped to manage their finances in the second half of their life.

If you know how to add, subtract, multiply and divide, you are fully capable of taking your finances into your own hands. To me, personal finance revolves around making sure you have enough money when you need it and not having sleepless nights fretting about difficult conversations with your bank manager.

Whatever money or income you have to live on, your goal is to be realistic about how much you need and to budget accordingly. If your needs are greater than the money you have available, you are faced with the following options: get a job, work more hours, find a better job, or sell your home and downsize, thereby giving yourself a lump sum to live on. You do not want to end up in the final decades of your life not being able to live as you would wish. Money matters now more than ever because you are planning for your future, which, by the way, could be a lot longer than you think! Make it a priority.

If you think I should not have included a chapter about finance, think again. According to a report released by the Prudential Insurance Company, two-thirds of pensioners living in poverty are women. The report also suggests that this imbalance could worsen. In fact, the annual average pension for women retiring in 2010 is at least £7,000 less than the average man's – £12,169 for a woman and £19,595 for her male counterpart. Three in ten women over the age of 40 admit that they are relying on their partner's pension for income in retirement. Considering that half of all marriages end in divorce, and over half of these divorces occur when women are over the age of 45, taking a punt on your future security by not learning, understanding and ultimately mastering your finances is not only risky, but stupid.

Mr Micawber almost had it right. Having enough money may not bring happiness, but it does bring peace of mind. When big changes happen in your life, how you manage your finances becomes even more important, particularly if you have recently divorced, lost your job or become widowed. The purpose of this chapter is to give you some tools to proactively manage your financial life.

How to manage your finances

No matter how much you have, money is one of the biggest issues in everyone's life. We live in a consumer-driven society where having just one of something is not enough. More is not only more: more is better. Very few people think they have enough money, but millions think they don't have enough. When money becomes tight, it can create horrible feelings of instability, insecurity and fear. Life is simply much more expensive than we think it is.

Money is usually less of a problem if you and/or your partner are employed. It only becomes an issue if you divorce, your partner dies or you lose your job. One of the most common misconceptions amongst divorcees is that they expect to live the life they did when they were married. With only half, or less than half, of the previous income to live on, this becomes virtually impossible to achieve. If your income is insufficient and you are not working, go and get a job. If you haven't worked for a while, keep reading. The next chapter is about how to get the best job you can. In the meantime, there are things you should be doing now to make the most of the money you have.

As you start to plan for the years ahead, you must answer this apparently simple yet complex question: how many years do you need to plan for? Although the official life expectancy for the average 50-year-old woman in the UK is currently 82, there are new studies that indicate this number is too low. Professor Sarah Harper of the Oxford Institute of Ageing has recently suggested that a healthy 50-year-old woman can now expect to live until 96, and a man to 91. This means you could have over 40 more years of life still to fund.

Realistic planning is important because it allows you to accurately assess where you are in your financial life. Below are six key questions that you should be able to answer with confidence:

1. What are your annual expenses?

2. How much debt (mortgage, credit cards, etc.) do you have?

3. What are your sources of income (job, pensions, ISAs, life assurance, savings, etc.), and how much income do you generate in a year?

4. Are you likely to inherit money or divorce or retire?

5. Do you own your home? What portion of your net worth is in this single asset?

6. Have you and your partner written a will?

1. Annual expenses

Whether you are well-off, on a pension, still working or retired, you probably spend more money on essentials than you realise. Working out a budget for now and the future is a good way to create peace of mind. Review your cheque book/credit card bills to get a sense of one-off expenses (home, car, holidays, children, other family members and elderly parents) and try to gauge what those might be going forward. Cash flow is the key to making ends meet. If you can properly assess what your expenses are, you will have a realistic idea of any surplus or shortfall. Let's look at those expenses one by one and see what they should include.

EVERYDAY LIVING

Food, eating out (don't forget to include your daily cappuccinos from Starbucks!), clothes (how many handbags and shoes do you buy each year?), dentists, doctors, health insurance, travel (buses, tubes, taxis), cigarettes (give them up now!), alcohol, mobile phones, toiletries, make-up, daily newspapers, magazines, subscriptions, birthday gifts, etc.

HOME

Mortgage or rent payments, council tax, maintenance and repairs (painters, plumbers, electricians), gas, electricity, water, oil, building and contents insurance, phone bills, PC maintenance and repairs, printer paper and cartridges, etc.

CAR/S

Cost of replacement, petrol, servicing, road tax, insurance and repairs.

HOLIDAY/S

How many holidays do you take? Flights, hotels, meals, spending money, insurance, gifts and souvenirs.

CHILDREN AND OTHER FAMILY MEMBERS

Food, clothing, holidays, books, iPods, iPads, mobile phones, school fees, nursing care (and other extraordinary expenses related to ageing parents and other family members).

OTHER EXPENSES

Credit card interest, books, jewellery and life insurance. A big expense that you might not have budgeted for but could need to in the future is private health insurance. Patients are increasingly turning to the private sector for routine procedures, such as hip, knee, hernia and cataract surgery, because of 'rationing' and long NHS waiting lists. If you don't have private insurance, a typical knee replacement will cost you around £7,000.

A SMALL EXPENSE TO ADD TO THIS LIST

Saving and filing all your receipts but not keeping proper records does not qualify as keeping track of your monthly expenditures. If you do not know how to use a Microsoft Excel spreadsheet program, take a one-day class or purchase a book or DVD to teach you. This will help you to keep proper tabs on your expenses and may be one of the best investments you can make towards balancing your budget.

2. Debt

Mortgages are about the cheapest way to borrow money and credit cards are the most expensive.

MORTGAGE LOANS

The way most of us got onto the property ladder was to take out a mortgage. Although mortgages are one of the cheapest ways to borrow money, they are still a debt that needs to be repaid. When you were in your 20s or 30s, you still had 30 or 40 years of income-earning potential ahead of you to pay that debt, but as you head past your 50th birthday, your income-earning years are limited. Unless you want to sell your house to pay off your remaining mortgage, reducing it should be your priority.

Over the years, many people have asked me how they should invest a lump sum that they have inherited from their parents or a relative. My advice is always, 'Use the money to pay down your mortgage.' The maths are easy. If you are paying 6 per cent on the loan and your tax rate is 40 per cent, you need to get a pre-tax return on any investment of 10 per cent to equal the return you get by paying down your mortgage.

The last time I came across an investment product that guaranteed a 10 per cent return was in the 1980s when interest rates were high. This brings me to an important point. Do not forget that mortgage rates can go up sharply and in a very short space of time. You probably remember the early 1990s, when mortgage rates hit 15 per cent. Do not be complacent and expect them always to be as low as they are now. Can you afford to pay your mortgage if interest rates go up to 10 or 12 per cent instead of 5 or 6 per cent?

If you are looking to make money the easy way, pay off your mortgage. There is no better guaranteed investment return.

CREDIT CARD LOANS

If you can borrow money any other way than by credit card, you should. Why? Because a large percentage of credit card borrowers default and cannot pay their bills, and this pushes up the interest *you* pay, which can be 3–5 times more than traditional lenders charge. The typical interest rate you will be paying, even in a very low-interest rate environment, is over 20 per cent per annum. You will become the gerbil on the wheel, running to stand still. It is financial suicide. Always try to pay your credit card bills on time.

Don't attempt to save money in a savings account until you're out of debt. Any interest you pay on your debts will more than cancel out what you make on your savings, so net–net, you are effectively losing money, not saving it. In fact, according to data from Bloomberg financial analysts, if you live in the UK, the money you keep on deposit is now losing in real terms – 4.6 per cent per annum, or £460 on every £10,000 of savings! A scary thought for anyone living off their savings.

If you're in a situation where you have many credit cards with outstanding bills, you should investigate consolidating them onto one card. Shop around to get the best interest rate and you could make substantial savings. Your monthly payments will be lower, and closing your other accounts could improve your credit rating.

3. Income and savings

Know what all your different sources of income are and budget accordingly.

YOUR JOB

For most of your adult life, you and/or your spouse will have worked, and your income will have paid for your lifestyle. As you enter the second half of your life, you will need to think about how to support your lifestyle if you can't work because of retirement or health issues. If you are divorced, you will need to think seriously about whether or not you should go back to work or look for a higher-paying job. Perhaps in your current job, you should be asking for a pay rise, working more overtime, applying for a promotion or taking an additional part-time job. Take an evening class that teaches personal finance, investing, marketing, leadership or computer skills to help get a better job.

PENSIONS

When we were young, the idea of saving for our far-off retirement had little or no interest. In fact, when I asked several 25–40-year-olds if they'd thought about a pension, they responded with, 'Pensions are stupid' or 'It's 40 years away' or 'Why would I want to save for a pension that will be worthless by the time I need it?' All these opinions are misguided. It's in your best interest to know about pensions long before you need to draw on them.

According to the 2010 Scottish Widows Women and Pensions report, older women are not saving adequately compared to men of the same age. Women aged 51–59 have accrued on average only £37,642 in retirement savings compared to £54,345 saved by men. This report also highlighted that women's own private pension savings for retirement are still well behind men's – in fact, 35 per cent of women of working age do not even have a pension scheme compared to only 22 per cent of men.

There are three types of pension.

- **State pensions** is a regular payment people can claim when they get to State Pension age. Once you get your State Pension, it gives you a regular income for the rest of your life. You should be aware that the government has announced new proposals for increasing State Pension age. For both men and women it will rise to 66 by the year 2018. Almost 22 per cent of all women are depending entirely on the state pension for their income. You can get your forecast by going to the government website www.direct.gov.uk/en/Diol1/DoItOnline/DG_4017970).

- **Company pension** is a pension scheme set up and administered by a company for its employees. It may be contributory – with employees making pre-tax payments direct from their salaries – or non-contributory, in which case the company makes the payments on its employees' behalf. There are two types of company pension schemes:

final salary – or defined benefit – schemes offer pensioners a proportion of their salary at retirement; or defined contribution schemes, whereby the risk of poor investment performance – or untimely decline in annuity rate – lies with the individual pension holder.

- **Private pensions**, also known as personal pensions, is when an individual pays a regular amount, usually every month, or a lump sum to the pension provider who will invest it on their behalf. The fund is usually run by either a building society, bank, insurance company or unit trust. If you are self-employed, not working, or work for an employer who does not offer a company pension sheme, a private pension may be a suitable vehicle for you.

Many women do not have a clear idea of their financial situation, with four in 10 women who *do* have pensions not understanding how they work. If you haven't done so already, you need to spend time thinking about how much money you have saved in your pension plan and the number of years you have made National Insurance contributions. There are ways to increase your contributions while you are still working. If you have paid off your mortgage and the children have moved out, review your finances and see if you can afford to pay more into your pension.

If you don't get your state pension forecast figured out, you are forgetting to tick an important box. This forecast can help put the amount of money you will have in retirement into perspective, as it also works out your likely expenditures in the future. This is a wake-up call to help you realise the true cost of retirement and whether you can afford to do it.

Keep your eyes open to the years ahead. You do not want to wake up at 75 years old and realise you have run out of money. Be realistic about your prospects, budget carefully and cherish your savings. You will need them.

A pension is not your only option to build up money for the long term. Other ways include savings accounts, ISAs and other types of investment. (Your home may be the largest investment you have.) Each type of saving and investment works differently and has its own pros and cons.

ISAS AND LIFE ASSURANCE

If you have any savings or investments, you should have an ISA (Individual Savings Account) set up. The reason? It is another way besides a pension that you can save or invest tax-free, thereby increasing your returns. And you can have instant access to your money without losing the tax benefits on what remains in your ISA.

It may also be worth considering life insurance, also known as life assurance, as a safety net. If your spouse dies, it will provide you with a lump sum that can help pay off debts. Look for life assurance that does just that – cash value life assurance.

Do not be tempted by life assurance that sells itself as a savings plan. Most of these policies sold by insurance companies have had poor investment returns as a large amount of the premium you pay ends up in salesmen's commission and helps the insurance company with their overheads. Seek a financial adviser you trust and who will charge you fairly.

HOW TO FIND A FINANCIAL ADVISER

The first thing to be aware of is that many independent financial advisers (IFAs) are paid on commission, or a fee and commission, or salary bonus and commission. The salesmen who are selling you their products to 'help' you, are measured by how much business they do and by the commissions they generate, not by how much money they are making you.

With this in mind, try to find an adviser you trust, who is smart and will work on a fixed fee or for a fixed percentage of assets. Ask friends who they use, or someone who you think is smart and good with money. Your solicitor may also be able to make a recommendation. You can also find independent advisers at the big banks too. Ideally, you want to make sure they are being paid only by you and not by the firms whose products they might recommend. Of course, none of this guarantees a good return, but at least you know you are getting objective advice.

My recommendation is to interview two to three advisers to get a better sense of the different approaches that can be taken. Most people don't know how to do financial planning, so you actually need someone in whom you can have confidence. You must feel comfortable that you are both on the same page with the same goals.

Remember the lesson. Know how your adviser is incentivised. This means you need to figure out how they are getting paid. Always ask questions if you don't understand something. It is your money and you have hired the adviser to help you. You don't always have to agree. Listen to what is said and then make your own decision.

4. Retirement, divorce and inheritance

For most mere mortals there is little choice whether to work or not. Early retirement is not an option. The question is rather how long one can stayed employed, not how soon one can stop working.

You know my view on early retirement. Don't do it. And now the government doesn't want you to retire either. It will make you old before your time. However, it is important that you map out your predicted income and expenses as outlined above well ahead of the time when you finally decide to stop working.

DIVORCE

Becoming newly single again can put many women in a panic scenario, especially about their finances. When interest rates were 8 or 10 per cent, the income generated by a lump-sum divorce settlement was frequently adequate to support a divorcee. Today, with interest rates below 1 per cent, this is not the case. If you are in the process of getting divorced, please bear this in mind. It might be better if you get your former spouse to guarantee you an inflation-linked annual payment in addition to a lump sum, rather than looking to maximise the lump sum itself.

I have several friends who were awarded what looked like a generous lump sum but no income, and who are now eating into it at a rapid rate as their capital is generating no income. For emotional reasons many women settle for the family home and give up their right to their husband's pension. Again, this is dangerous, as many find they have neglected their own retirement needs.

You should try to negotiate for a participation in your ex-husband's future income growth. What is the point of being married to someone for 25 years, then finding a year after you divorce that his new business venture, which he was working on for the past six years, has finally taken off?

If you don't understand the world of money and have convinced yourself you don't have any interest in learning about it, you need to get yourself reoriented. Becoming better informed by taking a class about finance or getting appropriate advice will be a good first step in your journey to banishing your fears. Make the time to build your skills. Knowledge is power.

INHERITANCE

If you have inherited money, your goal should be to hang on to it. Do not speculate with it. Whoever left it to you spent a lifetime working for that legacy. Unless you are very wealthy and can afford to take some risks, any lump sum inheritance should be used to help pay off your mortgage. Have I made myself clear on this yet?

You should also consider setting some money aside as a 'disaster fund' for emergencies. If possible, you should have enough cash in a bank to live on for six months. This is how you will manage if you get sick or lose your job. It is financial suicide to have your money tied up in a way that you cannot access some immediately.

With the interest rate environment being so low at the time of writing, it is impossible to find an investment vehicle that both provides income and allows capital to grow at least in line with inflation. When interest rates start edging up again, seek professional advice. A good place to start is at your local high-street bank. Your bank manager can be surprisingly helpful when it comes to maximising interest on your savings account.

5. Home sweet home

As we grow older, we don't have as much flexibility in how we spend our money. Most of our expenditures are predetermined at the beginning of every week. Budgeting is the name of the game, and you might find that you simply don't have enough cash for your spending needs.

Asset rich and cash poor is not a good situation to be in during the second half of your life. Chances are you are living in your biggest asset. What portion of your net worth should be in your home? By selling your home and downsizing you are solving several financial problems at once. You will be lowering your monthly maintenance costs, council tax and utility bills, and giving yourself a lump sum for a rainy day.

6. Your will

Whatever your financial circumstances are, please make sure you write a will. As it is a legal document, it needs to be done properly, so you will need a lawyer. You will also need to select an executor – someone who will ensure your final wishes are carried out.

Your will can specify everything from what you want your funeral to be like to who should receive your treasured belongings. You don't want your relatives squabbling over who gets which piece of jewellery or the car. More importantly, do you want your relatives to get everything? Would you like to leave something to one of the charities near and dear to your heart, which you have been spending time helping in the past few years? What about your godchildren? Your cleaning lady who has worked for you for the past 30 years?

Spend some time thinking about who and what you want to include in your will. One only has to flick through various glossy magazines to see how the children of wealthy families are giving meaning to their lives. The rule of thumb is that if you are the first generation to make some money, the next generation will spend it and by the third generation it is completely gone. Parents who tell their children that they will inherit money are doing them a grave disservice. Children who are waiting for their parents to die to inherit their wealth are living an unrealistic existence. Their parents will be living longer and need the money.

Our generation could be the first to be living with four generations of family, so think long and hard about how much money and in what time-frame you want your children, grandchildren and great-grandchildren to receive it.

Inherited money can really screw up the next generation – their core values, motivation, entrepreneurial spirit and the basic business of living a productive life. Then again, according to Virginia Woolf, 'it was her fuel for intellectual and artistic creativity'. Be careful. When it comes to inheritance, less is more.

Risk

Risk needs to be considered in everything you do in life. Picking a husband or partner, allowing your kids to go on public transport at night, learning to ski, walking down a dark street alone, smoking, not exercising enough and how to invest your money. How well you manage your risk will determine how successfully or unsuccessfully you negotiate your way through life.

Would you be willing to risk borrowing from or lending money to a friend or family member without considering the effect it might have on your relationship? By clearly documenting how you will pay back or lend the money, you are protecting your finances and one of the most important relationships in your life.

I spent 20 years of my professional life working in finance and ended up running the equity business of a public US investment bank in London. There was a lot of pressure to produce revenues because we were all judged by how much commission we generated. You could be the smartest person in the City square mile, but if you didn't produce the goods, you didn't keep your job for very long.

My husband and I have many friends who ended up using their savings or a lump sum inheritance to speculate in internet and other technology stocks towards the end of the technology bubble, thinking it was a savings account, only better. Do not be fooled; with any investment comes risk.

Investment 'truths' that are just wrong

- **Residential property always goes up.** Need I say more?

- **Equities always go up in the long term.** The love affair has been over now for some time.

- **You need lots of life insurance.** You only need life insurance if you are likely to have an inheritance tax bill.

- **I never charge a fee.** Everyone charges. Know where the hidden charges are and what that charge is as a percentage of the assets that you are investing.

- **You can't lose.** You *can* lose money in anything and everything: property, commodities, equities, bonds.

- **All banks are the same.** They are not. JP Morgan and HSBC have been very safe, while Northern Rock and Anglo-Irish Bank were not.

- **Certain investments are like having cash.** Over the years, many financial instruments having an enhanced return have claimed to be cash or nearly cash. It is only cash if it is cash. Nearly cash doesn't count; it is called an investment.

Personal finance: not a game of chance

Widows, single women over 50 and elderly couples are viewed as easy targets for people selling investment products. We are viewed as unsophisticated and at the bottom of the food chain. The products they want you to buy are the products where there is excess capacity. You need to spend some time making sure you are not throwing your hard-earned money away. It should not be like betting on the horses or hoping your number comes up in roulette. Never pass on or take a 'hot tip'. 'Hot' has a way of turning frigid by the time it gets around to most of us.

Of course there are plenty of financially savvy women who can run their family finances. But when it comes to investing, I think this group becomes much smaller. Even the men and women who are at the epicentre of finance and have access to the best money managers around the world know that there are huge risks involved in investing. Some of the best brains in finance have ended up losing the bulk of their money.

When I retired from finance in 1999, I decided to invest a bit of money for our children in 'younger growing companies' that I thought could be the next Microsoft or Apple Computer. Eleven years later, I can report that 80 per cent of the stocks I chose have grossly under-performed. So be careful. If you can't afford to lose money, don't invest it.

My top 10 tips

1. Know where your money is. How is it invested? Who is it invested with?

2. Know your rates of return and the income generated from your capital. Always consider the impact of taxes. Make sure you are thinking in terms of after-tax money when considering rates of return.

3. If you can find an excellent adviser who you trust, it is worth the money you pay him or her. Make sure you understand

how your adviser is paid. Remember to go in with your eyes open and interview two or three.

4. Know how much your life costs to run today. It is fundamental to your future. Calculate what your income will be when you retire. Figure out your priorities, what is essential and what you value in your life and work. Basic maths: if the money coming in isn't covering your bills, you have only two choices: either reduce your expenditure or increase your income.

5. Remember that life expectancy is going up with every year you live. Add in at least 10 extra years when you are working out how you are going to maintain your standard of living.

6. Never risk any money you can't afford to lose. If you can afford it, better to give it to a charity and have the pleasure of knowing you are helping an organisation or cause that you care about than have to suffer the pain of watching your capital either completely disappear or dwindle to a fraction of your original investment.

7. Other than your home, do not have all your eggs in one basket. You need to spread your risk no matter how safe the historical track record of that basket might seem.

8. Assume you can get a better deal on your utility, phone, car and household insurance bills. Spend time shopping around every year and the savings could be substantial. Check the fine print to know how long you are committing yourself to any new contract. While you're at it, if you rent, be aware of what other rentals cost in your neighbourhood. You might find the same-size flat around the corner for £100 less a month.

9. If you can afford to pay down your mortgage, use your money to do so.

10. Pay off your credit cards each month. Even with lowest-rate credit card, there are far less expensive ways to borrow money.

When you learn more about money, it will become less of a burden and possibly something you enjoy. Although the Beatles wrote a hit song based on the belief that 'Money can't buy you love', money goes a long way in bringing peace of mind, relieving stress and making life a lot easier. By understanding and learning about finance, you give yourself the chance to have enough money for the things that bring you pleasure in the second half of your life. Having just enough money to stay connected to family and friends, exercise almost every day, eat nutritious food, live with purpose and cultivate at least one passion in your life will mean you have given yourself a platform to continue to transform your life for the rest of your life.

CHAPTER FOURTEEN

Going back to work
Preparation equals confidence

'Because I am a woman, I must make unusual efforts to succeed. If I fail, no one will say, "She doesn't have what it takes." Instead they will say, "Women don't have what it takes."'

Clare Boothe Luce, writer and US Congresswoman

If you are a woman who is working and enjoying her career, feel free to skip this chapter. If, however, you are not happy in your job, or you are thinking about going back to work because your children are older, this chapter will provide you with a good road map for how to go about the process of getting back to work and landing the best job you can.

Have you worked most of your adult life in a job where you felt you used only five per cent of your brain because it was more important to have job security and more flexible hours so you could pay the bills and be around to raise your children? Or are you one of the many intelligent, highly accomplished women who chose to give up the day job in the middle of your peak earning years to be at home to raise your kids? Now that your children are older, you are ready to use some of the extra bandwidth that has become available in your brain. Perhaps your new post-menopausal brain is urging you to explore your own creativity and re-engage with the world in a new way?

Let me warn you now – finding the right job will not be easy. It will require reflection, soul searching, research, courage, commitment and possibly going back to school to have the career you want. You are ready to take the necessary steps to make these dreams a reality. It is as if a switch flipped, a light went on, and you are now ready. You are feeling re-energised and have come to the realisation that 'Now is my time'.

You are not alone. You might feel alone, but you are part of a large and growing number of women either returning to work after the age of 50 or who have never stopped working and want to use these next decades as an opportunity to make the most of your years and qualifications. In fact, according to the Department for Work and Pensions, by 2020 a third of the UK workforce will be over the age of 50, and women will account for 80 per cent of the workforce growth. Aviva Life's Real Retirement Report (2010) revealed that over 50 per cent of women see working well past retirement age as a viable option to keep them from having to spend an additional 7.5 hours a day with their spouse!

At this moment, you might not be sure how to make your goals a reality, but you know there is an ember burning inside you that is ready to ignite this passion alongside the desire or need to make some money. For some, this process will seem like starting from scratch. Whether it is writing a new CV, networking, applying for a new job, being interviewed or negotiating your salary and benefits package, the process is daunting – especially at this time in your life.

Returning or rethinking?

Are you well-educated but haven't worked for a while? Just fed up with the job you have and want a change? A McJob is not what you have in mind. You don't want to work just to work. You want the start of a career. You want your work to combine passion *and* a pay cheque. Ideally, you would like to find a job that blurs the line between work and play. Can you leverage the time you've spent working in the community for free into a paid job? Can you turn a passion, such as gardening, cooking, painting or design, into money? Or do you need to go back to school to retrain for the career you want?

Women who have never worked or didn't work long enough to have a 'profession' believe career women learn a 'secret language' in the office. This secret language comes from years of working as part of a team, being recognised for doing a job well, and giving and getting respect from co-workers. After a while, the confidence this generates becomes second nature in the way you make decisions and work in a group. You know how to 'talk the talk' because you have been speaking this language for years.

This experience gives working women a springboard to confidently approach what needs to be done in their lives. It is similar to a muscle memory in sports. Working and having a sense of achievement becomes part of who you are. You think you can do anything you put your mind to. Working gives you a skill set that can be applied to everything you do in your life. It will also give you the psychological safety net when things are not going well in your marriage, with your bank manager, or even with the van driver when he is two hours late with your grocery order. You have an innate sense of how to turn things around and make them work. Granted, you might not always succeed, but the self-belief is there.

If you haven't worked for a while, or you have been in a job that didn't exactly challenge you, this doesn't mean you can't learn how to talk the talk and act the part. Years away from an office or working in a job that bored you does not mean you cannot apply your skills to what you want to do next. However, you must know what you are talking about, and to do this requires preparation.

Top tips for returning to work after a break

These tips come courtesy of Annita Bennett, co-founder of the executive search firm Taylor Bennett.

- Make sure that all your domestic cover, from childcare to cleaning, is well established, with back-ups where necessary. You will already be concerned about the impact of returning to work, and this will allow you to worry less when you finally do. If you have a partner, discuss the impact of changing patterns on life at home.

- Work out your mental salary base so that you know your minimum market price before considering any opportunities that come your way.

- Find professional friends or approachable headhunters to dissect your first attempts at a CV. This is your first and only sales tool ahead of an interview, so it needs to be *au courant,* professional and human. Be happy with the final version, as it will be your basic interview script.

- Use the best of those who helped you with the CV to give you a practice interview. You will be nervous about presenting yourself, unclear what to emphasise and unfamiliar with discussing salaries, so these sessions will calm you down and reduce 'first-interview-for-years' nerves.

- Buy two outfits that look great and will work in the professional environment. Don't forget shoes and bags. You will suddenly feel as if you are ready for the part.

- Read the *Financial Times,* the *Economist* and any other papers or websites whose opinions you respect so that you feel up-to-date before launching yourself.

There is a logical process to finding the right job, whether you want to change jobs or re-enter the workforce. It is the preparation and the hours you are willing to put into this process that will ultimately determine how successful you are in your quest.

Sometimes you have to figure out what you *don't* want in order to have the courage to go after what you *do* want. Below are a dozen basic steps that will start you in the right direction.

1. Think about what you want to do. This is the time to define or redefine what you want to do and the working life you want to create for yourself. Ask yourself some obvious questions:

- Do I want a temporary, contract or permanent job? There will be pluses and minuses to each, but you will need to figure out what type of work you are looking for.

- Is the company conveniently located for my life? Realistically, how long are you willing to commute every morning if you are not prepared to relocate?

- What kind of company do I want to work for? Small, big, multi-national? Public or private sector? Would you like to work for a charity or not-for-profit organisation?

- Will the company offer any training? Will there be any opportunity for career progression? Are there good healthcare benefits?

- Would this company be a good fit for me? Do your prospective colleagues seem like people you could get along with?

- Have you thought through the pros and cons of starting your own business? Have you done enough research to analyse if there is a need for your new business idea? If lack of money is the issue, you don't want to lose your shirt before you even get started.

- Can you afford to go back to college, or could you take a job where they offer you the training you need? Should you use the skills and the work experience you had before you stopped working to get a good entry- or mid-level job and work your way up the ladder?

2. Take a career test. This will help you to realise what your innate strengths and weaknesses are. The tests, such as the Myers-Briggs or the Birkman, are professionally administered and reviewed. There are also free personality/psychometric tests on the internet (do an online search for 'best tests to find a career' and 45.7 million hits come up). If you can afford to, seek professional advice. You would never dream of getting divorced or writing a will without a lawyer, and I think the same professional approach is needed for career transitions. A career counsellor or life coach can advise you what your strengths are and how to leverage them, and to make the most of your education, work and volunteer experience.

3. Write a basic script to sell yourself. Before making any phone calls, you must know exactly what you are going to say: what you are looking for, what skills you have, and what you bring to that particular type of job. Nobody will know unless you tell them. You must be prepared. Writing out the entire script puts you in control of the conversation. Have your key bullet points ready to fall back on at any time during the call. Remember, they can't see you. This is the phone-in part of the process. Practise on your husband, partner, best friend or children. Figure out exactly what you want to say and how to say it quickly. If you can't say what you need to say in the first two minutes, keep re-editing your script.

4. Start networking. Women are complete naturals at connecting all the dots and making things happen. Knowing how to ask questions and having the confidence to request help will save you endless months in your job search. If you are still friendly with former co-workers, bosses and teachers, it can unearth surprising results. Talk to people you have met socially, perhaps through your children's school. Call anyone and everyone you know who you think might be able to help. It is often the people you least expect who come up trumps.

Kate Grussing, founder of Sapphire Partners, a pioneering consultancy firm dedicated to getting professional women back to work, believes that men and women approach networking very differently. 'When men network, they think of it as a trans-action. He calls his friend at the company he wants to work at and says, "Joe, would you set up an interview for me?" Men want to get the deal done. It is matter-of-fact. Women don't tend to do this. They might call the same person and say, "Do you know of anybody who might want to help me?" Or "Would you like to have a coffee? I need your advice." Of course, women get there in the end, but just not as quickly.' Kate's advice is for women to try to be more direct. Ask and ye shall receive!

As part of your networking, talk to employment agencies and executive search firms, research industry organisations and use the web. Professional websites, such as LinkedIn, Xing and Spoke, can direct you to the right organisations and people. So can industry associations, such as the Media Society (PR) and the Association of Chartered Accountants (finance), while others, such as Professional Boards Forum (www.boardsforum.co.uk), can put you in touch with professional women. Don't forget that your college or university alumni association can also link you up with old friends and possibly useful contacts.

Executive search firms and networking groups, such as Sapphire Partners, Taylor Bennett, Women Like Us and Women's Business Forum, work with professional women who have taken a career break and are looking to begin working again, or with women who are looking to advance their careers. Research which companies are committed to hiring older workers in your area, take advantage of government training schemes, and remember the non-profit sector for job opportunities.

5. Write a new and convincing Curriculum Vitae (CV). Your CV is really the first piece of paper a prospective employer will receive about you when you apply for a job. It is essential to get it right. It will improve your chances of being selected for interview and getting your foot in the door. You must spend time making sure your CV reads the way you want it to. There are standard formats for CVs and I would recommend you refer to the Reed Specialist Recruitment Agency website (www.reed.co.uk/careertools) to help you create one.

This is definitely a case where less is more. Your CV should be one page only. I don't care if you were a governor of the Bank of England, one page should say it all. With one page, the parts of your life that you want to highlight will stand out. It needs to be concise, typed in a simple font (Times New Roman is a classic and very readable), and there should be sufficient spacing so you can actually see the different section headings. After your name, address, email, phone number and date of birth come the headings: Education, Work Experience, Board and Volunteer Work, Additional Skills or Talents, and finally your Hobbies or Personal Interests.

At a glance, a prospective employer should be able to garner your key skills and experience to determine if you should come in for an interview. If you've taken any evening classes or enrolled in further education, please include details as this shows you have determination and curiosity. Remember, each of these entries should be concise and to the point. Don't emphasise dates unless you think it will benefit you.

If you have any additional skills or talents, such as fluency in a foreign language or IT skills, be sure to include them. A woman I spoke with decided to interview for a job in the development department of the British Library. Although she hated the idea of raising money, she always loved books and wanted to work in an environment where she would meet other people who shared her passion. Instead, she was hired as a translator because under Additional Skills in her CV she had put 'Ancient French', and they actually needed someone to translate books in that language. She hadn't worked for over 20 years and was hired for her dream job!

Remember to include one sentence at the bottom of your CV about your hobbies and personal interests. These might include tennis, theatre, dance, medieval and Renaissance art, modern ceramics, Pilates, yoga, cooking, ping-pong, backgammon, gardening, quilt-making, reading to schoolchildren, your book club, swimming or travel. It matters because it tells the interviewer something special about you. During my years in finance, I once had a CV come across my desk where a woman listed theatre, particularly musicals, as one of her personal interests. I decided to interview her because she had similar interests to mine. Her CV stood out because she loved the theatre but wanted to work in finance. Your hobbies and interests should give a glimpse of who you are and your personality. When interviewers aren't sure what else to ask, they will inevitably ask about something you enjoy doing. Make sure you include this on your CV.

The head of an executive search firm mentioned to me in passing, 'Most men will embellish their CVs and bios without any qualms, while women will tend to downplay their achievements.' Make sure you know what you want to say and make yourself sound like someone you would want to employ. Remember, if you can convince yourself you are the right person for a job and can articulate this, you are actually doing a prospective employer a huge favour. You are helping them to solve their problem.

6. Write a thoughtful covering letter. This is an important part of the application process because it gives an opportunity to make an impression, and emphasise your skills and experience for the job in question, while making reference to your CV. Ultimately, this means that a good covering letter will make the person perusing it take a bit of extra time to examine your CV. It also means you have a much better chance of being granted an interview. Covering letters should be kept short and to the point: no more than three paragraphs before signing off.

If you are re-entering the job market after many years, your covering letter provides an ideal opportunity to explain why you want to go back to work, what your strengths are, and any skills you picked up along the way. If you have been introduced to the company by someone in the company or a friend of the person interviewing you, mention this in the first paragraph. If you speak another language fluently, this is your time to high-light it. If you chaired a charity committee or a brilliant fundraiser, include this too. IT skills should be mentioned, but if you don't have any, you should seriously consider taking a course so that you aren't disadvantaged. Judith Kark, principal of Quest Business Training College, says: 'Older women need a certain level of IT skills in order to compete in today's job market. They need to become computer savvy.'

7. Get any written references you can. If you haven't worked for a while, you will need to ask the chairperson of the local volunteer organisation you worked for, the head of the PTA or the principal of your children's school to write you a reference. Although this is one of the most important things on your 'to-do' list, it isn't for the person you are asking. These things always take a lot longer than you think, so remember to ask early and often.

8. Preparation, preparation, preparation … did I mention preparation? Of course, going to an interview and having to show the best of yourself in an hour is stressful. Add on top of this years of not working, or years of working in a job where you felt undervalued and under-utilised, and you could be a nervous wreck. Are you worried that you will be older than your new boss? Are you worried you will be viewed like a mother hen? Take a deep breath.

Before any interview, you must ruthlessly research the industry and the company and have at least three intelligent questions to ask. You should be able to give five clear and good reasons why you are the right person for the job and be able to articulate them in less than two minutes. Chances are that the person you are trying to convince will have made up their mind about you in the first 45 seconds. The less time it takes to convince someone of your suitability, the more successful you will be. Preparing what to say will give you confidence, but you must make sure you actually say it. Do not assume the person interviewing you has memorised your CV. Speak clearly and give your interviewer the important and relevant information. Do not say anything negative about yourself, your life or even the weather! Please remember to repeat important points.

You want to radiate confidence. You will show that you have thought not only about the job you are applying for, but also the company you could be working for. If you prepare properly, you will subconsciously be saying, 'I know who I am. I know who you are. I have researched your company and the job, and I am the person you want to hire.' It is critical you are able to convince a prospective employer that you are bright and articulate, ready to show initiative but also someone who respects authority. You need to exude confidence so your prospective boss will listen, trust, respect and hopefully do what you want them to do – hire you! Creating a successful outcome involves believing in and knowing how to sell yourself.

9. Look the part. Even if everyone else in the office is wearing jeans, being slightly overdressed is a million times better than being underdressed. You want to look as if you will fit in, so clothes should be well tailored and blend into the background. Remember, modern classics, such as the white shirt, the blazer and the sleeveless A-line dress, can look a lot more professional and a lot less ageing than the black bondage look.

10. Speak with authority. During an interview, the following question always comes up: 'How would you describe yourself?' A good response is, 'I asked a few friends this question over the past few weeks as I was trying to figure out what I would be best at and in what direction I should focus my skills and talents. I was pleasantly surprised by their answers. They described me as [choose three] adaptable, organised, positive, trustworthy, confident, thorough, friendly, hard-working, innovative, proactive, reliable, responsible and smart.'

The next question will undoubtedly be: 'What would you say is your worst trait?' Please, please, please do not use this as an opportunity for a mini therapy session. The only response to this question should be something to the effect of, 'I can be too much of a perfectionist' or 'I am an overachiever' or 'I am a complete workaholic as soon as I get involved in a project. My husband wonders where I get my energy and drive from!' Those are your only answers!

Do not talk non-stop. You will appear desperate and undesirable. Do not say that getting this job will solve your problems. Do not laugh unless someone, either you or the person interviewing you, has actually said something funny. Nervous laughter shows a deep-seated insecurity. It is easy to do this when you are nervous, but remember, answer the questions thoughtfully and directly, then shut up or ask the interviewer one of the brilliant questions you prepared.

11. Send a follow-up letter or email in the next 24 hours. There is nothing like a heartfelt letter emphasising how your skills and interests would be a perfect fit for this position.

12. Know approximately what you are worth. The question of salary might not come up until you've been offered the job, but then you need to know what the job will pay, and what you need financially to make it worth your while to go back to work.

Most companies are old-fashioned when it comes to hiring women who stopped working. Swallowing your pride and accepting a lower salary to work for the right company with the right working hours, the right amount of travelling, and the right opportunities will be important factors in making your decision. However, you do not want to feel cheated or that they are taking advantage of your situation. Never refuse or accept a salary straight away. You should always give yourself time to consider all your options.

If the salary is on the very low side of what you were expecting, and you are not compensated by either career development or additional training, you will need to face the fact that this job is probably not for you. Don't despair. Stay positive and keep networking. Remember, most jobs are not advertised.

If the salary is close but not enough, ask if there is any flexibility on the amount offered. Also ask how often this salary is likely to be reviewed. If it is going to be reviewed regularly, this could make it more acceptable to you. If there is no flexibility on the money, you might ask them to reconsider the benefits package. Although it is not money in your pocket today, it might offer fantastic healthcare coverage, a generous pension, bonus incentives, or flexible working options.

If you like the company, its culture and the people you met during the interview process, if you think you will enjoy the job and there is room for career development, be realistic and willing to take a lower starting salary to get back to work or change to a job with more scope and upside. Working gives you a lot more than just a salary. It creates an environment where you can create strong new social connections and find purpose and new meaning.

Back to school?

Whether you want to pick up where you left off or start a new career, going back to work in your 50s or 60s might mean going back to 'school' first to get further qualifications. Start thinking ahead now. You need to have a plan. As one woman told me, 'I started to plan this next stage of my life in my mid-40s. I knew if I didn't that I would vegetate.' For many women, going back to school is a great way to re-engage, and is ultimately the stepping-stone to going back to work. You might even meet your next business partner or employer while furthering your education.

This is a time to merge your passions and interests with an income. Working in a job you enjoy will give you financial peace of mind, while keeping your brain active and your outlook positive, confident and optimistic. Ultimately it is the belief in yourself, your ability to identify both what you are good at and what truly interests or inspires you that will make working in the second half of your life work for you.

CHAPTER FIFTEEN

Old is the new old

Redefining old

'It's a different stage of life, and if you are going to pretend it is youth, you are going to miss it. You are going to miss the surprises, the possibilities, and the evolution that we are just beginning to know about because there are no role models and there are no guideposts and there are no signs.'

Betty Friedan, author of The Feminine Mystique

We only have to look at the last hundred years to appreciate the fundamental changes that have happened to women in the West. If we think back to our grandmothers, who had the trials and tribulations of living through two world wars, they had no choice but to take whatever life dished out. It was an endurance test. Life was about survival and continued existence. Many spent the majority of their fertile adult years pregnant, giving birth or lactating. Many died in childbirth or lost their children to disease or in battle. A 40-year-old woman was considered old; a 50-year-old ancient. Getting older definitely meant becoming less empowered.

Our mothers were born in the transitional period between two kinds of society, two economies and two philosophies. They lived through the Great Depression, which was followed by rising standards of living. They were more vocal and aspirational than their own mothers. Our mothers grew up having the right to vote. Advances in both science and industry changed forever the way they lived. Our mothers raised us with luxuries: refrigerators, cookers and televisions. They listened to music and had opinions about rock 'n' roll, films and fashion. They saw the first man walk on the moon. Although life was easier, women were still confined by the boundaries of their time.

Our mothers never articulated their inner voice. They were encouraged to confine themselves to a very narrow definition of womanhood that directed all their energies to making their husbands happy.

There was no place in the world they lived in to voice unhappiness or discuss the changes happening to their bodies. They were expected to endure in silence, pretend they were not experiencing any hormonal symptoms and carry on as usual. I thought about calling this book *What My Mother Should Have Told Me*, but that would have been unfair. Our mothers and grandmothers did not have the choices or opportunities to redefine what it means to grow older.

Swept away by the wave

Change for women of our generation began in the 1960s, with the invention of the contraceptive pill, which allowed them to make responsible choices and decide whether or not to have children. In 1963 came the publication of Betty Friedan's book *The Feminine Mystique*, which exploded the postwar myth that homemaking was everything for a woman. Friedan called it 'the problem that had no name'. Friedan declared that if you weren't fulfilled by polishing floors, making beds, trying new recipes and giving up your dreams, there were other possibilities to find satisfaction. Marriage and children did not necessarily equate to happiness and sexual fulfilment, the same way that pursuing a career did not mean a woman was destined to spinsterhood and celibacy.

An exploding population, advances in labour-saving devices, feminist legislation, a belief in equal rights for all, and courageous women who fought for equality – in the home, in the bedroom, in the workplace, in education, in politics and in government – challenged everything our mothers believed in their pursuit of a new prosperity and the dreams of suburban living. The youth-focused sexual and cultural revolution soon followed. Our generation, the baby boomers, were swept away by a new wave of feminism. This really was the dawning of a new world order.

> We are the first generation of women comfortable enough to articulate our *inner* voice. We will become the wise women in our villages as we define successful ageing.

The fourth wave?

What does this mean? Feminism as a radical movement has come and gone. The first wave, in the late 19th and early 20th centuries, revolved around political power and the right to vote. It shook society to its core. The second wave, from the 1960s to the 1980s, was about equality and radical change: breaking the glass ceiling, equal pay for equal work, equality in marriage and the importance of sexual satisfaction. Nobody is really sure what happened during the third wave, which emerged in the 1990s, because there was no single doctrine. It was more about women defining feminism for themselves.

Today we don't really know what being a feminist means any more. Of course, many of us relate to the goals of feminism, but we do not identify as feminists. Why should we? Women in the Western world are doing nearly everything men do, and more. We still don't get equal pay for equal work, and there are not enough women in positions of power, but today there are more women than men working in America. By 2013 the UK workforce will mirror that statistic.

Gloria Steinem, the American feminist and founder of the magazine *Ms*, once said, 'We will never solve the feminisation of power until we solve the masculinity of wealth.' And we know this is coming soon too. The female consciousness is alive and well and an organic part of our culture.

Could accepting and rejoicing in the second half of our lives – breaking pre-existing stereotypes and redefining what it means to be old – be the long-awaited fourth wave of feminism? Could this fourth wave be a reflection of what happens to the female brain after menopause – a fusion of understanding and acceptance, a desire to push outside our traditional boundaries and create a new place for ourselves in the world? Could this be the time when women can finally be who they want to be and answer to themselves while continuing to be intelligent, challenging and maintaining the essence of their femininity?

Not only do I think this is possible, I think it is probable. Women over 50 are becoming a bigger part of the population with every passing year. In both absolute and relative numbers, we are not alone and we are not invisible. According to the Office for National Statistics, men and women over the age of 50 comprised 34 per cent of the UK population in mid-2008. Over the next 20 years, this number will be trending towards 40 per cent. Logically, how can there be a stigma or a silence to ageing if we represent a large and growing percentage of the population?

The meaning of age is definitely changing. No longer is there this huge gulf as we move through our 40s, 50s, 60s and 70s. Depending on the choices we make, an 80-year-old can be functionally younger than her 50-year-old daughter. Ageing is now a continuum from middle age to old age. Women who clearly celebrate being over 50 are our new role models: they inspire awareness while sharing an 'ageless' ability to get what they want from life, and have an endless energy for curiosity, self-discovery and re-creation.

Radical change isn't easy, but it can happen. After World War II, and simply through sheer numbers, the baby boomers created a demographic bulge that transformed Western societies. All the children born in the West between 1946 and 1964 were considered to be part of this generation.

We were a product of choice and change, and grew up genuinely expecting the world to improve with time. If you were born during this period, you hit the jackpot. In fact, there was no better time to be a teenager, a 20-year-old, a 30-year-old or a 40-year-old, because we were the ones creating and then redefining the ideological and cultural shifts that occurred in the world. I believe we continue to live in the sweet spot of life, and there has never been a better time to be a post-menopausal woman.

What exactly are advertisers trying to sell us?

Advertisers still have a retro-engineered fantasy about the over-50 market, despite the massive demographic transition that is reshaping countries, economies and markets, the reality of the population shift is that the pyramid has inverted, with the ageing baby boomers at the top and today's youth at the bottom.

When I wrote my first article about the joys of menopause, it was for a national weekly magazine. I suggested to their new editor that my article, which was to become the cover story, would be a perfect vehicle to sell advertising. I thought she was listening because a couple of days later she called, absolutely thrilled, as she had sold numerous pages of it. However, it was to the manufacturers of incontinence products, stairlifts, portable bathtubs, walking frames, raised toilet seats, lift-assist cushions and magic bras!

The advertising industry has not yet realised that we, as a generation, are dictating a new cultural shift. We are buying mountain bikes, iPads, iPods, Kindles, computers, cars, trainers, exercise gear, holidays, work clothes, health-club memberships, designer shoes and handbags. And we are buying more than ever before.

It makes me think of the line in the film *Pretty Woman*, when Julia Roberts returns to a shop in Beverly Hills where she was previously considered to be an inappropriate customer. Now armed with dozens of shopping bags from other stores on Rodeo Drive, she says to the sales assistant, 'Big mistake!' It is time for advertisers to realise that it is the over-50s who are buying their products, and that we aren't particularly inspired by the 18-year-olds advertising them.

Old is the new old

In the same way that we have put our stamp on every decade we've lived through, we will, once again, speak with one voice our new philosophy about this stage of life beyond middle age. Old is not the new young; 50 is not the new 30; and 70 is not the new 50. *Old is the new old.* The spirit of this statement requires a mindset that believes we can break pre-existing stereotypes and attitudes in order to age in a way that makes sense for the world we live in. If the opportunities we look for do not exist, we need to create them.

We know we don't want to age like our mothers or grandmothers, but nobody ever showed us or told us *how* to age. In the past, it was expected that women should, at a certain age, simply step back and watch the world go by. We now know that this is a recipe for premature ageing in every dimension – physical, mental and spiritual. We have begun and will continue to make conscious choices not to become trapped in a downward cycle of ageing. Just as we influenced politics, education and the economy like no other generation before us, we will unite in the second half of our lives to shape new ideas and put ourselves in a position to help each other and our community.

❝ There is a special place in hell for women who do not help other women. ❞ *Madeleine K. Albright*

Mad men and angry women

The 1950s marked a difficult time for both men and women. Not only did women lose their sense of purpose after giving up their work outside the home during the war, but men were handed what they thought at the time was a golden parachute – forced retirement. On paper it sounded like the deal of the century: the freedom to do whatever they wanted and get paid for the pleasure for the rest of their lives. In reality, this provided men with the bona fide chance to lose the core of their lives and the structure necessary for human connection and purpose. They were simply not ready for the 'what next?' and were effectively forced to grow old before their time.

Rethinking retirement

There is no historical precedent for the number of men and women alive today who are over the age of 65 – not just alive, but full of vitality and ready and able to continue making a difference to society. Past generations would start work at 14 or even younger and die at 65. They lived in a labour-based society in which life was defined within the parameters of employable years. Today there are few jobs in which the intensity of physical labour or mental skill warrants *any* retirement age. We now live in a knowledge-based economy, where the only movement is the moving around of information.

Although the current government has now proposed a 'no mandatory retirement age' policy to be put into effect by the end of 2011, there is still a great need to rethink and provide opportunities to reflect the fundamental shift in the demographic structure of our society. Could government and business work together to create incentives to keep the ageing population working longer, encourage recruitment, retention and the retraining of the ageing workforce, all to create new policies to reflect the world we live in?

Is the 40-hour working week a sacred cow that cannot be touched? Could government change the way that an employer pays National Insurance after the age of 65 so there are incentives to keep the ageing population working? Could government initiate a higher tax threshold on the first £15,000 of earned income so it would be tax-free for those people who continue working over the age of 65?

What has become clear is that the retirement of a productive person with years of wisdom and experience to a life they have not chosen is detrimental to the individual and to society as a whole. But we will change this too. Our generation, the now-ageing baby boomers, will drive new ideas and policies because our generation was empowered with hope and nothing got in our way.

> We grew up believing our voice made a difference because it *did* make a difference. We had a golden youth. We did not have to fight a major war and we had every reason to believe we would have a golden future.

We will work together to figure out how to redistribute opportunities and all the possibilities that come with them. We will drive new ideas and policies about the realities of growing older that make sense for the world we live in now. Old age is no longer a period of ill health, instability and closing doors. It is a time of staying fit, eating well, rediscovery, having self-worth and a purpose greater than ourselves.

Talkin' 'bout my generation

We had the loudest voice. With this voice we empowered ourselves and we benefited from freedoms that did not previously exist for women. We were the 'me' generation, and with that came the rise of the self. We came up trumps. We forged ahead at home, at work and in politics. We broke the glass ceiling, made traditionally male careers ours too, earned our own money, had our own definition of sexual freedom, and created more economic and personal freedoms, while benefiting from improvements in healthcare, technology and a higher standard of living.

We are the golden generation. This belief did not belong to our parents and it does not belong to our children. As we age, we carry this mystique with us. We will use our voice and the strength of our numbers to change the prevailing wisdom about how to age. This will be our greatest gift to ourselves and to future generations – the gift of personal choice. We will consciously choose how we want to live the second half of our life.

This is not about making seismic changes to our lives. This is about making a few minor changes to reap rewards hard to imagine at this moment. Part of this is taking responsibility, engaging with society, enlarging our circle of concern and making a difference. To do this we must make informed choices about how we want to live for the next 30 or 40 years and make conscious decisions about how to share our wisdom with the world around us. We are in uncharted territory because there are no rules in place about how to redefine and reframe this time in our life.

If we build it, they will come

It is my hope that integrated health and social care centres will be established over the next few years to help women manage all aspects of their menopausal life. Under one roof, nutritionists, physiotherapists, psychologists, gynaecologists, endocrinologists, pharmacists (to formulate and dispense individualised hormone treatments) and career and benefit advisers would serve as a 'one-stop shop' to serve the needs of older women. These centres would be a place where women could share their concerns and openly discuss their menopausal years for what they are: a natural part of life, not as a disease or illness that needs to be 'dealt with' or swept under the carpet.

From small acorns grow great oaks. The seeds of change have already begun to take root. It is my hope that our generation of women will come to celebrate the years after menopause as the beginning of a new and prolific phase of life. The gift of menopause is that we now have the confidence to begin again and the mindset to stay committed to this journey for the rest of our lives. By making passion and purpose our *raison d'être*, connecting with friends, family and our community, and exercising and eating well as part of our daily life, we will teach by example what growing older means.

The revolution is not over yet

When old is synonymous with active, strong, vibrant, courageous, soulful, creative, talented, determined, connected and life-affirming, 'old is the new old' will mean we will not fear the second half of our life any more than we did the first half. This new age revolution is coming and we will once again change the world.

CHAPTER SIXTEEN
Women to women
Guiding principles
to share

'Reflecting on your own life, what advice would you give other women to make the second half of their life the best half?'

Acting

'I don't really feel in a position to give advice to women about the second half of their lives because I never had children. I think the years when women raise their children define them. That said, I have been incredibly lucky to have found acting, a profession that I love and am able to grow old doing. I suppose the one piece of advice I could give to other women, no matter how old or where they are in life, is never be afraid to try new things or discover a hobby or a purpose that you feel passionate about. This will completely change your attitude about growing older.'

Dame Eileen Atkins, actress

'Basically, don't panic. Think up rather than down. I think the attitude tends to be "I've brought up my family, I've had my children, I've looked after everybody, and now what am I going to do?" And so many women I meet think it's about waiting to die, literally! Well, it isn't. It's about spending the time between now and when you do die fully and to the max, doing everything you've never had the chance to do, so that when death does finally come, it's a bit of relief to sit down and have a rest! And I'm not being frivolous about that. You know, there's nothing we can do about getting old, there's nothing we can do about death. What we can do is embrace the years that we have left to the greatest possible degree. So banish fear, anxiety and "What if?" Get up every morning and think, "Right – when and how?"'

Lynda Bellingham, actress

'I have always tried to be as brave, compassionate, strong and confident as I can be, and to meet all those nasty little surprises head on. And to laugh – a lot!'

Cherry Gillespie Dickins, actress and former dancer with Pan's People

'I remember when I was in my teens, my mother said, "Oh, wait until you're over 50 – it's wonderful!" And she was right. You don't have your periods, ambition has settled down, you don't have all the boyfriend problems, you can study (my mother took a degree when she was over 50), you know how to say no, and you know what you want. And there are just so many things that are better. Your children are grown up. Some people are divorced and very happy about it. And grandchildren are just amazing. So there is lots and lots to look forward to. And also, when you're young you're always worrying about your appearance: are your bosoms this, are your thighs that, is your hair whatever? When you get older you don't care: you just enjoy being older. The wrinkles don't matter. They're just a kind of proof that you're wiser and older and have enjoyed life more.'

Susan Hampshire, actress

'If there's one piece of advice that I would give to women about the second half of their life, it's probably the same as for the whole of life. It's a Quaker saying: 'Live adventurously'. And the good thing about the second half of your life is that you have more freedom to do so because, hopefully, you'll not be still entirely responsible for your children. Your grandchildren will be around, but they're not entirely your responsibility, so suddenly you have this *amazing* freedom to do exactly what you like and to be *utterly* selfish. For example, I have an utterly selfish car. It's a sports car, a two-seater, and if anybody chooses to come with me they *cram* into the back and I don't care because I've had vile people-carriers all my life and I'm enjoying my sports car.'

Sheila Hancock, actress and author

'Turning 50 has been *great*! After feeling so gloomy and doomy about the prospect on my 49th birthday, it has been a surprisingly uplifting experience for me. The new-found lightness and joy is mainly, I think, that I feel I am finally living in the present. Hurray!

'I have suspected for decades that in the struggle to find happiness, confidence and serenity – "living in the moment" – is the key, but how to realise this simple yet highly elusive concept? It seemed ever to escape me.

'I believe it took turning 50 for me to confront the brutal reality that I am well over halfway through my adult life and that unless I start to "do it now" (whatever "it" might be), it is probably never going to happen. Being 50 is a great boost to clarity, spirit and drive!'

Greta Scacchi, actress and activist

'The first piece of advice, without which the other bits become irrelevant, is to look after your health. Make sure your body is cared for and serviced like a car for as long and as comfortable an onward journey as possible.

'Break old habits. The good ones will stay with you, the bad ones haven't worked. Discard them. New habits bring new perceptions.

'Open up to people of all ages. Unlike young people, you know what it is like to be young, middle-aged and old. You can relate to everyone.

'Befriend your older appearance. Don't deny it or try to recapture your young looks with surgery. There is a way of being beautiful at every age.

'Imagine every year is your last and try to do as many of the things that, on your deathbed, you would regret never having done.

'If you are lucky, like me, to still be working at 60, don't lose your thirst for a challenge until you drop.'

Harriet Walter, actress and author

'My advice would be to get over yourself. Whatever you've achieved, everyone's forgotten about it already, so the only person you have to answer to is yourself. And if you can look in the mirror and say, "Boy, am I getting more interesting!" then you've accomplished something. I always wanted to show my parents that I was really smart and to be able to say I went to Oxford. So that's what I'm doing now. It's really nothing to do with the second half of life; it has to do with there being things I need to finish before they put me in the ground. I would like to be a model too, but I think that's probably first-half material. Going to Oxford will feel like I'm being taken seriously and that I'm covering the whole range. My epitaph won't just be, "She was a funny girl, she was a comedienne, she was an alcoholic." I'd like to cover the whole spectrum. "She was an alcoholic, she was a comedienne *and* she went to Oxford" – that would be nice on my grave.'

Ruby Wax, comedienne, author and facilitator

The Arts

'Make the most of every opportunity and every second. Don't put off anything you've dreamed of doing, whether it's work, travel or something you wish you'd done when you were younger – studying for a degree or learning another language. Time is precious and races by when you get older, so don't waste it – every second counts. It's better to die fulfilled, having achieved your goals and aspirations.'

Janice Blackburn, curator and art critic

'Don't let menopause trip you up. It doesn't have to change who you are. I more or less ignored it. Find something that you are passionate about and immerse yourself in it. For me, love of family, meeting people, travel and my obsession with making pots keep me energised.'

Jennifer Lee, potter

'The real answer is a noxious combination of caffeine, alcohol and prayer. (For this read: Please, God, don't let me strangle my daughter when she acts like Linda Blair.)'

Elsie McCabe, director, African Art Museum

'One must never stop learning or laughing. I never want to stop being nosy ... whoops, I mean curious.'

Nicola Reed, artist and Kitchen Round Table member

'Now that I am over 60 years old, there is nothing better than the excitement and challenge of a leadership role that combines my passion for the arts and for education.'

Debbie Swallow, director of the Courtauld Institute

'Find what feels true and beautiful to you, to your own true nature, and follow where it leads you. Honour your own truth.'

Emily Young, sculptress in stone

Athletics

'Run your own race. Try to keep living your dreams and follow your heart. I recently went to Chicago to celebrate the 25th anniversary of my fastest marathon by running another marathon. Couldn't miss the opportunity to run on 10.10.10.'

Joan Benoit Samuelson, first woman to win
the Olympic marathon

Authors

'For me it is a combination of luck, good genes and a love of reading that has taken me through a wonderful second half of my life. Nothing more.'

Diana Athill, editor, novelist and memoirist

'My advice is to go on growing. It's a big mistake to assume that because you've passed 50 the best is gone and it's downhill from now on. Fifty might not be the peak. It might just be the foothills. The important thing is, whatever has happened so far in your life is leading forward to something important. Go on growing. Extend your friendships. Widen your interests. Travel, start a new hobby ... Try something different. Wear different clothes. Try out different make-up. Have a good time. Read different books and magazines. There is absolutely no end to what you can do.'

Dame Joan Bakewell, author and broadcaster

'1. Don't just love your children, enjoy them! And if you don't, set about repairing the rift as fast as possible. There's nothing sadder than seeing two adults (mother and son, mother and daughter) who don't get on. However great your career, children are the most precious things in life.

'2. Keep fit, which sounds boringly predictable, but is oh, so true. I broke my leg when I was 52 and spent 20 months on crutches and sometimes in a wheelchair. It was a taste of what being really old might feel like, and I want to keep that at bay for as long as I can. Not being able to run for a bus makes you feel vulnerable in whole new ways. So hang onto it and do yoga.

'3. Keep colouring your hair for as long as you want/can. It's very cheering.

'4. Learn something new every year. I now work in the government, a whole different career from life in the media. It's brilliant for keeping my brain cells alert and interested. I love going to work.

'5. Love is just as good and just as bad at 60 as at 18 and, I suspect, as at 80. So never give up.

'6. See your girlfriends and go on holidays and trips with them.

'7. If you're married, make sure you have your own life without the involvement of your partner. They might drop dead at any time.

'8. For the same reason, always have your own money.

'9. We are not our mothers. We're the baby boomer generation, who have been inventing our behaviour since we were born. The truth is, there are no longer any rules attached to ageing, so it seems like a great idea to enjoy the fact that you're wiser, less likely to panic about things that really don't matter, and to love the fact that we live in a time where we can still work, love and learn right on until the grave.

'10. Forget what you ought to do (you've been doing it all your life) and do what you want to do.'

Rosie Boycott, journalist and feminist

'This might sound corny and obvious, but *be yourself*. The great Miles Davis used to tell young jazz trumpet players, "It takes a long time to be yourself", and it does. Life never stops being scary and strange, and that's good. Keeps you on your toes. Lately, I've discovered that I'm actually too young to do certain things, like wear mini skirts, for example. If I'm lucky to have another healthy 20 years, that's for my 80s! Right now I stay as healthy as I can, but don't overdo it: no Botox, no facelifts, no heavy make-up – but I don't put down the women who do.

'Also, I don't criticise or envy or emulate young women. That's the worst, especially for us baby boomers, because we should know better.

'I let young guys treat me with respect, and have a great time (and much sympathy) for older men. In other words, I continue to be as I have always been, but even more so.

'I call myself an "old lady", although I know that many women don't like that term. But I was lucky to grow up around older women who were loved, respected, fancied, looked great and took no guff off anybody. So being an old lady was always a goal. They're cool.'

Bonnie Greer, playwright, author and critic

'Work hard. Love well. Give back. And above all, and as often as possible, have fun.'

Katie Hickman, author

'Set your goals impossibly high. After all, you now have the experience and the wisdom to achieve anything you set your mind to. And be sure to make your goals meaningful ones that match the values and beliefs you have developed over the first half of your life. There is still time to change the world!'

Lisa Jardine, historian, author and broadcaster

'Don't have cosmetic surgery. Just let a man read between your lines. My mother told me never to pick my nose, especially from a catalogue. Dimmer switch, girls – greatest sex aid known to womankind.'

Kathy Lette, author

'I think it's a time to get really curious about yourself and your reactions to things because you've lived a lot, you've accomplished a lot, you know a lot. Now it's time to look afresh and see what you don't know, and what you might need to know in a different kind of way.'

Susie Orbach, author and psychotherapist

'Never give up. You are still you with valuable layers of experience added.

'Give love, time and energy to family, friends and new projects.

'Try not to be scared by the fast-changing world; join in.

'Your enthusiasm will make you a role model for daughters and granddaughters.'

Eve Pollard, journalist and broadcaster

'Look ahead, never look back. Embrace everything and be grateful.'

Carol Rocamora, author, playwright and educator

Charity and fundraising

'In the second half of my life when my mother died and my husband died and the kids went out of the house I found myself, suddenly, absolutely alone and lonely. I had to fill my life, which led me to introspection on the spiritual journey but that still was not enough. I had to embrace my entire life. I did not have to belong to just one family, mine, but to consider the entire world, everybody, as part of my life. That gave me the purpose to live from minute to minute.'

Tara Gandhi Bhattacharjee, Vice Chairperson,
Kasturba Gandhi National Memorial Trust

'After learning at age 52 that I had been misdiagnosed and had stage two melanoma, my life changed in so many different ways. The frightening reality that I had a 50 per cent chance of my melanoma metastasising and that there was no cure was an extremely powerful call to action. With four wonderful children, I faced the sickening realisation that I might not be lucky enough to watch them grow to adulthood.

'Melanoma research has become my mission, and I have thoroughly immersed myself in a whole new world of science and cancer research. Each day I know I am able to help make a meaningful difference so that people do not suffer and die from melanoma. I also live each day knowing how very lucky I am to be able to enjoy my life.'

Debra Black, co-founder Melanoma Research Alliance

'Know, believe in and love yourself, and everyone else will too. Listen to your gut feelings – they are almost always right.'

Catherine Faulks, Conservation fundraiser and
Kitchen Round Table member

'Count your blessings. Notice the many things that are working, whether a relationship, a body part, the hoover, the car, the taps or your internet connection. No matter what your challenges, you can be absolutely certain that there are plenty worse.'

Ingrid Jacobson Pinter, chairman, Kensington & Chelsea Volunteer Bureau and Kitchen Round Table member

Design

'Maintaining a good level of fitness, eating healthily, working hard at something you truly love and taking time for yourself each day is my mantra for retaining an inner strength and discipline that ultimately leads to a richly rewarding life and well-being.'

Tricia Guild, designer

'Now that I am 50 I have relaxed into being myself. I realise that the stress of seeking the approval of others is unnecessary. I have accepted that I am naturally eccentric!

'I try to instil confidence in others, as I feel that this is the key to living happily and successfully. I live life a day at a time and know that laughter is often the best medicine.'

Lulu Guinness, designer

'I grew up in Iraq in the 1960s and, as in so many places in the developing world at the time, there was an unbroken belief in progress and a great sense of optimism. The ideas of change, liberation and freedom of this era were critical to my development.

'It is very important to have the commitment to persevere, and to go back to one's own education in a sense. As a woman, you need the confidence that you can carry on and take new steps every time. I truly believe in hard work; it gives you a layer of confidence. For a period in the mid-1990s we did one competition after the other – and we didn't win any. It devastated us, and I had to pick up the pieces, but they were all great designs; very powerful projects and interesting in their complexity. I'm fundamentally an optimist, and I knew I would eventually come out of that situation. You have to adjust your thinking every once in a while to fit the moment.

'I'm always curious about the next step – the next big thing. With every period there needs to be an exciting new challenge.'

Zaha Hadid, architect

'There is a wonderful feeling of liberation associated with the second half of one's life. You have choices. You can decide. Take a little time for yourself. It's your turn! And as long as you don't abuse anyone else's agenda, friends and family will support you.

'Celebrate your intolerance! Never confuse it with being difficult or cantankerous. It comes as a direct result of your own previous experiences either at home or in the workplace. And experience really does count.'

Betty Jackson, fashion designer

'My best advice at any age is to try to understand the world we live in. Go to art galleries, museums (free), concerts (£7 at the Barbican). Read. This is all completely relevant to your present life. The present is always the present moment of the past. The past is what we are. Modern propaganda has been against this. Instead we have been told to keep up with the times – and consume (including opinion).

'Get off the consumer treadmill. Spend less, yet have a more interesting life – active, not passive. You get out what you put in. You will have a sense of personal progress.

'By engaging with the past you engage with the present. All those points of view from people who think differently from us will make you start to think.'

Dame Vivienne Westwood, fashion designer

Directing and producing

'I like to keep my mind on the goals so that obstacles don't stop me from moving forward. I like to look for and find humour in everyday occurrences. Feeling that I have something to give people now and in the future is what continues to make life fulfilling for me. I love knowing that I can make a difference to better humanity even in the smallest way – that if I give a smile, I can create a smile in others.'

Marsha Lee, director, screenwriter and
Kitchen Round Table member

'I think the great thing about the second half of one's life is that you've had so much practice at living that you're really quite good at it by the time you get to the age of 50. And all kinds of things that felt really, really hard and really, really frightening in one's 20s, 30s and 40s suddenly feel "Oh, here comes that moment again". And there's a certain kind of "cashing in" I think, of experience, that makes life really fun. There were all kinds of things I was told would not be possible after the age of 45, such as falling in love and finding a new partner. Well, I can say that's untrue. I was also told that if I hadn't directed a big feature film by the time I was 40, it would never happen. Wrong. I did.'

Phyllida Lloyd, theatre and film director

'Try to be more curious than afraid. And never miss an opportunity to laugh at how ridiculous life can be – and how genuinely funny, too.'

Marla Rubin, theatre producer and Kitchen
Round Table member

'Education, education, education and role models were key. They were tools to discover and develop our talents, and to see it's okay to aim high. We all need to find that touch-paper inside to really take off. We must teach our daughters to be bold and brave and to take risks. I want to carve out calmer time, to enrich my own life of the mind, but also find space for simple pleasures, such as gardening, spending more time outdoors to really appreciate the seasons, travelling, cooking, sharing, talking, arguing with children and grandchildren and friends and any young women who will listen. Life is rich and beautiful. My best advice is to keep working to achieve your potential, while balancing it with time to enjoy many life's simple pleasures.'

Rosemary Squires, co-founder and joint CEO,
Ambassador Theatre Group

'If you want to have a glittering post-menopausal career, get your menopause in early. Mine started (without asking permission) at age 46, so I had plenty of time. I'd spent my early years as a radio and TV producer and presenter, but many wonderful things came together in the second half of my life. It wasn't until the hot flushes had subsided that I produced my first feature film (with Gerard Butler), went to Hollywood for my first Emmy nomination (for a TV movie starring James Woods) and co-produced my first West End play (starring young heart-throb Josh Hartnett). All of which proves that sheer tenacity, doggedness and experience can pay off if you just hang in there long enough.

'Of course, there are important life lessons to be learned along the way. One is that nothing and no one is perfect, not even you. *Especially* not you. So if you want to stay in the career game (and to be a good team player), keep reminding yourself that whoever said "Don't let the perfect be the enemy of the good" had a point. (PS: This also applies to your marriage or partnership.) Reminder to Type A personalities: cut everyone some slack.'

Jane Walmsley, film, theatre, TV producer and author

'Keep active. Do not obsess about ageing. Try to love your ageing face and feel proud of what you have achieved. Keep your brain occupied with different projects. Have a lot of friends of different ages and interests. Think about what brings you happiness and ensure that it features in your life. For me it is music and theatre. Ensuring they are part of my life means that I meet a lot of talented, wonderful people.'

Hilary Williams, theatre producer and
Kitchen Round Table member

Education

'Find an activity or cause that impassions you – sporting, cultural, intellectual, spiritual – and build it into your life; fit other appealing but less compelling activities around it. Make sure to exercise regularly in whatever way works for you, and make time for social networks and friendships. Finally, keep meeting new people and trying new experiences so that you will stay challenged and stimulated.'

Nancy Broadbent Casserley, design historian and
Kitchen Round Table member

'The focus shifts from acquisition and defining oneself in the traditional ways to tuning into the larger community. How can you make a small positive mark on your world? (The concept of "the world" is rather too big an undertaking!) How can you find meaning in the world beyond the confines of the family, which is where one's focus tends to be for so many years? Find something that could benefit others from your gifts. Give back. The endless focus on self needs to change and to embrace something bigger.'

Julie Horowitz, educator and counsellor

'Embrace the sense of empowerment that being on the other side of the menopause can give you, if you let it. I have felt stronger and steadier, and better equipped emotionally and temperamentally for the cut and thrust of public life.

'I would say that my relationships have led to my success and happiness. As a youngster, I don't think I was conscious of this. I thought they were all down to hard work, ambition, focus, positive thinking, etc., but almost as soon as I started working at a City law firm, I felt that it was an empty achievement to be a partner and never see your family in any sustained way. So what has made me and continues to sustain and develop me is the secure foundation of family. The other ingredient of my happy life is fulfilling and absorbing work – in the broadest sense.

'My advice is give more than you take and the rewards are huge.'

Marianne di Giorgio, educator, counsellor and
Kitchen Round Table member

'Being hopeful and having faith that things will work out has kept me moving forward. At 48, with two boys aged 16 and 18,

I became a widow when a truck hit my husband while he was jogging in Las Vegas on a business trip. We never said goodbye. Getting over that was slow, but five years later I am remarried to a fabulous man, reconnected with my most precious friends, and have a great job.

'I believe that having daily goals have made my work and life easier. Life is good when you open to it. I can't see where the entire second half of this life will lead, but one day at a time, riches are being unearthed.'

Felice Shapiro, Professor of Entrepreneurship,
Tufts University, Boston

Homemaker

'What makes life fulfilling? My children, my family, my friends, the ballet, my tennis, the theatre, opera, movies, books – but mostly people and making them smile.'

Peggy Post, mother, grandmother and charity fundraiser

Industry and business

'During the second half of your life, there are fewer urgent pressures from raising a family and building a career. My advice is to actively choose how you spend your time. Spend more time with those wonderful friends you have made over the years. Make sure you are available to spend time with your children. They now have lives of their own, and you need to be sensitive to their busy schedules and fit in with their priorities. Spend the morning talking to your husband over a cup of coffee.'

Judy Bollinger, Chairman of ABG Sundal-Collier,
Philanthropist and Member of the Kitchen Round Table

'By the age of 50 few of us have managed to dodge having to face our worst fears: serious illness, death of loved ones, divorce, bankruptcy, addiction. We have overcome, though we may be a little battle-worn. We are reinforced by our experiences, enriched by our friendships and are, hopefully, a little wiser. The freedom that comes with knowing you can deal with most of life's trials is indescribable. My mantra has been "accept and be free". Try it – it works a treat.'

Vanessa Branson, hotelier and arts patron

'Be true to yourself and try to seek out what you love and enjoy – always remembering that working as part of a talented team is better than trying to do it entirely on your own – and you will find success a lot easier to achieve.'

Melanie Clore, deputy chairman, Sotheby's Europe

'I have been most successful and happy when I have thrown myself into something – anything – completely. The confidence that you can make something happen; the belief that if you have faith in the right thing happening, it will; the enthusiasm that inspires other people to join you and follow you; the feeling of contentment that comes when you are 100 per cent engaged; the happiness that comes from achieving; all begin with your own willingness to get up, get going and be committed. Life is not a dress rehearsal!'

Diana Godding, financial consultant and Kitchen
Round Table member

'Everything I have achieved is due to four things: the values my parents instilled in me; the unconditional love and support of my husband and children; the loyalty of close friends; and the passion I have for what I do.

'Learn to stay open to everything that comes your way, and understand that all of it is a gift to help you grow and reach your next level of potential. The things that I resisted in the first half of my life created pain and disconnection, but when I look back I see how perfect that journey really was. So now I can relax, feel gratitude and truly relish and enjoy every moment of the second half of my life!'

Penny Mallinson, transformational consultant and
Kitchen Round Table member

'To solve your problems, first you have to acknowledge them, then you have to share them with those you respect. You will be amazed at the solutions that present themselves – even the ones you had already thought of! A fulfilling life is to challenge your-self to do your best in all your endeavours, and when you think you have fallen short, take responsibility. Rationalisation and self-justification are the antithesis of fulfilment.'

Norma Miller, restaurateur, author and Kitchen
Round Table member

'As I entered my 50s and the second half of my life, having achieved many of my goals in business, I decided to leave the corporate world and reawaken my creative side. I had a lifelong interest in photography, which I put on hold as I pursued my career, but recently I enrolled in a full-time degree course at the International Center of Photography in New York City. Trying something so new, so different, has been challenging, invigorating and scary. The most exciting thing is the knowledge that there is time in life for many chapters, for many careers, for many periods and for constant exploration. The critical part is staying engaged, connected to the world around you, continuing to learn and chal-lenge yourself, to take risks and to enjoy the journey. At the end of the day, you don't want to look back and have regrets.'

Hollis Rafkin-Sax, Vice Chairman, Financial Dynamics

'In order to make the second half of your life the best half, you have to believe that whatever and whoever you have been up to this point is only part of the story. Nothing has been determined and everything can change. Be open to that change and greet it with amused wonder. Every day, as I sit and read the material for my class, I wonder why, and then I just embrace the experi-ence for its own sake. No specific utility, there is joy just in the doing. That ability to live in the present only happened for me once the obligations of early family and career life were met. Be open and patient and good things will waltz in to your life.'

Gwen Snider, hotelier and student

'My advice would be always to try to think ahead. Be positive and face the worst, but project yourself towards the best. Take the steps to get there, but stay within your own personal morality to keep peace with yourself.'

Nicky Davies Williams, CEO, DCD Rights Ltd

Law

'Stay interested and you will stay interesting. Use these years to pursue the interests you had to defer during all those years of child-rearing and/or work. Learn a language; take an art class; study literature; immerse yourself in a history course. Resurrect old passions or find new ones. Give back; volunteer to help others by applying the skills you developed and honed as a mother and a career woman.'

Deborah David, mediator, lawyer and
Kitchen Round Table member

'Find your moral compass; live by it, and when you inevitably fail to follow it from time to time, acknowledge it and don't be bitter about the consequences. We all screw up occasionally.

'Family and friends are to be loved, nurtured and cherished. Without them, life would be a very dry husk.

'Don't be oppressed by the possibility of failure. A life without risk is not a life lived to the full.

'Trust your instincts and when they speak to you, follow them.

'Personal fulfilment comes in many guises. A life that is predominantly focused on achieving monetary success is unlikely to be a fulfilled life.

'Don't become a slave to your work.

'Laughter is the ambrosia of life.

'Thinking about this has made me realise that (for me) the key to a fulfilled life can't be summed up in a sentence or two.'

Melanie Hall, Q.C.

'1. Don't waste a minute. Get out there and do the things you love doing. People always ask me how I manage to do all that I do and I quote my mother who said: "You haven't seen her skirting boards." I learned on the job to manage my time well, and worked out what was unimportant, so I keep a good balance between work and play. In fact, I would advocate increasing the play element in the second half of life, especially with women friends. I also try to reduce drudge work to a minimum.

'2. Accept new challenges. I do so all the time and it means I keep learning, which is great, and I meet new, interesting people, especially ones who are younger than me.

'3. Cherish the people you love. Tell them how much they mean to you. Write it to them. Be expressive about it. I have experienced the loss of some of my closest friends and it reinforced my belief that we have to let people know how much our lives are enhanced by their friendship and love.

'5. Count your blessings. It sounds trite, but I look at my wonderful man and my children and I think how blessed I have been. Learn to shed bad experiences and move on. Holding on to anger or disappointment is time-consuming and diminishing.

'6. Celebrate everything. We have frequent parties, big and small, which give us opportunities to have toasts, pay drunken tributes and the chance to see our friends en masse.

'7. Take up yoga or Pilates or both. Staying flexible and learning not to fall over when you have to stand on one leg to put your knickers on is not a skill to be underestimated.

'8. Start giving things away – we don't need all this *stuff*. And do give away money. It can make such a difference to other people's lives, and it feels good.

'9. Before it is too late, choose an aspect of our world where you can make a difference by volunteering or contributing in some way. I try to do it around law reform, violence towards women and children, and making educational opportunities available to those who missed out first time round. The second half is a time to harvest what you know and put it to good use for real change.

'10. Make your bed one of the most comfortable places in the house and go there with your beloved in the afternoon whenever possible.'

Baroness Helena Kennedy, barrister,
broadcaster and educator

'My advice is to love well. It takes work and commitment, but it is oh, so worth it.

'Carry on learning. It feeds something you are passionate about.

'And keep laughing, because having a sense of humour is essential for making it through the bumps in life.'

Anne Fernald Niles, lawyer

Music

'The secret of a good second half is not to be afraid of what cracks you open because, to steal a great line from Leonard Cohen, "That which cracks you open lets the light in, and the best stuff comes out of the worst stuff."'

Beth Neilsen Chapman, singer/songwriter

'I never give advice to people! But the fact that I am fortunate to still be doing my work makes me a very fulfilled person. The most important thing in life is love, not just romantic love, but giving out positive and loving feelings.'

Petula Clark, singer

'Take a look and see who you really are and then accept that and try to make the change so that inner change happens too. I feel this is what gives you more of an enriching life because you're able to accept who you really are.'

Mary Wilson, singer and founding member of The Supremes

A final thought

There is a wonderful book by Jane Walmsley called *Brit-Think and Ameri-Think: A Transatlantic Survival Guide*, which supports what George Bernard Shaw once said: 'England and America are two countries separated by a common language'. As an American living in London since 1983, I have felt at times like I say to-mate-toe, you say to-mah-toe.

Over the years I have learned that French fries equate to chips, potato chips are crisps, an eraser is a rubber (this got me into trouble during my first month here!), the first floor is actually the ground floor and so forth. I can now add to this list the language of women, menstruation and menopause: a vagina is called a fanny, PMS equates to PMT, menopause is THE menopause, and hot flashes are hot flushes.

The fact that we use different language when it comes to menopause does not matter because all women share a common bond: if we live long enough we will definitely go through menopause. It is my hope that this book will provide a framework for women (and hopefully men too) to celebrate this time in our lives and help us overcome the obstacles that get in the way to become who we want to be ... finally.

Further reading

CHAPTER 1: SURVIVING OR THRIVING

Joan Anderson, *The Second Journey: The Road Back to Yourself*, Thorndike Press, Waterville, Maine, 2008

Ronda Beaman, *You're Only Young Twice*, VanderWyk & Burnham, Acton, Massachusetts, 2006

Louann Brizendine, *The Female Brain*, Morgan Road Books, New York, 2006

Nora Ephron, *I Feel Bad About My Neck*, Doubleday, New York, 2007

Sarah Harper, *Ageing Societies*, Hodder Education, London, 2005

Suzanne Braun Levine, *Fifty is the New Fifty*, Viking Books, New York, 2009

Sara Lawrence Lightfoot, *The Third Chapter*, Farrar, Straus & Giroux, New York, 2009

Christiane Northrup, *The Wisdom of Menopause*, Piatkus, London, 2009

Jaki Scarcello, *Fifty and Fabulous*, Watkins Publishing, Stamford, 2010

Abigail Trafford, *My Time: Making the Most of the Bonus Decades after Fifty*, Basic Books, New York, 2004

Anne Tyler, *Back When We Were Grownups*, Knopf, New York, 2001

CHAPTER 2: THE MENOPAUSE MASTERCLASS

Ivy M. Alexander and Karla A. Knight, *100 Questions & Answers About Menopause*, Jones & Bartlett Publishers, Sudbury, Massachusetts, 2005

Deborah Blum, *Sex on the Brain*, Penguin Books Australia, 1998

Dr Laura E. Corio and Linda G. Kahn, *The Change Before the Change*, Piatkus Books, London, 2005

Marilyn Glenville, *The New Natural Alternatives to HRT*, Kyle Cathie, London, 2003

Dr Marion Gluck and Vicki Edgson, *It Must Be My Hormones*, Michael Joseph, London, 2010

Jenni Murray, *Is It Me, or Is It Hot in Here?*, Vermilion, London, 2001

Northrup, op. cit. (Chapter 1)

Dr Robin N. Phillips, *Your Menopause Bible*, Carroll & Brown, London, 2008

Suzanne Somers, *Ageless: The Naked Truth about Bioidentical Hormones,* Three Rivers Press, Los Angeles, California, 2007

Suzanne Somers, *The Sexy Years: Discover the Hormone Connection,* Three Rivers Press, Los Angeles, California, 2005

Robert Wilson, *Feminine Forever,* M. Evans, New York, 1966

Pat Wingert and Barbara Kantrowitz, *The Menopause Book,* Workman Publishing, New York, 2010

CHAPTER 3: REGULAR EXERCISE

Jane Aronovitch, Miriane Taylor and Colleen Craig, *Get On It! Bosu® Balance Trainer,* Ulysses Press, Berkeley, California, 2008

Ed Burke, *Precision Heart Rate Training,* Human Kinetics Publishers, Champaign, Illinois, 1998

Adam Campbell, *The Women's Health Big Book of Exercises,* Rodale, New York, 2009

Canyon Ranch Staff, *The Canyon Ranch Guide to Living Younger Longer,* Simon & Schuster, New York, 2001

Chris Crowley and Henry S. Lodge, *Younger Next Year: A Man's Guide,* Random House, New York, 2004

Chris Crowley and Henry S. Lodge, *Younger Next Year for Women,* Workman Publishing, New York, 2008

Miriam E. Nelson, *Strong Women Stay Young,* Bantam Books, New York, 2005

Joan Pageno, *Strength Training for Women,* Dorling Kindersley, London, 2005

CHAPTER 4: DIET

Dr Susan E. Brown and Larry Trivieri Jr., *The Acid Alkaline Food Guide,* Square One Publishers, New York, 2007

Carole Caplin, *LifeSmart,* Weidenfeld & Nicolson, London, 2004

Dr Peter J. D'Adamo, *Eat Right 4 Your Type,* Michael Joseph, London, 2002

Jonathan Safran Foer, *Eating Animals,* Back Bay Books, New York, 2010

Rick Gallop, *The Gi Diet,* Virgin Books, London, 2005

Zoë Harcombe, *The Obesity Epidemic,* Columbus Publishing, London, 2010

Patrick Holford, *The 10 Secrets of 100% Healthy People,* Piatkus, London, 2009

James Levine, *Move a Little, Lose a Lot*, Crown Publishing, New York, 2009

Ian Marber, *How Not to Get Fat*, Quadrille Publishing, London, 2010

Paul McKenna, *I Can Make You Thin*, Bantam Press, London, 2007

Barry Sears, *The Zone: A Dietary Road Map*, Regan Books, New York, 1995

Michael van Straten, *The Little Black Dress Diet*, Kyle Cathie, London, 2006

Bharti Vyas and Suzanne Le Quesne, *The pH Diet*, Thorsons, London, 2004

Andrew Weil, *Healthy Aging*, Anchor Books, New York, 2006

Andrew Weil, *Eating Well for Optimum Health*, Sphere, London, 2008

Chapter 5: Looking your best without plastic surgery

Nina Gardia, *The One Hundred: A Guide to the Pieces Every Stylish Woman Must Own*, Collins, London, 2008

Lucia van der Post, *Things I Wish My Mother Had Told Me*, John Murray, London, 2007

John W. Roe and Robert L. Kahn, *Successful Aging*, Pantheon Books, New York, 1998

George Vaillant, *Aging Well*, Little Brown, New York, 2002

Chapter 6: Your changing brain

Tony Buzan, *Use Your Head: How to Unleash the Power of Your Mind*, BBC Active, London, 2010

Simon Baron Cohen, *The Essential Difference*, Penguin Books, London 2004

Katharina Dalton, *Once a Month: Understanding and Treating PMS*, Hunter House, Alameda, California, 1990

Charles Darwin, *On the Origin of Species*, John Murray, London, 1859

Helene Deutsch, *The Psychology of Women*, Grune & Stratton, New York, 1944

Thomas Gisborne, *An Enquiry into the Duties of the Female Sex*, 1797, University of Michigan Library, 2009

Lawrence C. Katz and Manning Rubin, *Keep Your Brain Alive*, Workman Publishing, New York, 1999

Ferdinand Lundberg, *Modern Woman: The Lost Sex*, 1797, Harper & Bros, New York & London, 1947

Susan Pinker, *The Sexual Paradox: Extreme Men, Gifted Women and the Real Gender Gap*, Random House Canada, 2009

Steven Pinker, *How the Mind Works*, Penguin Books, London, 2003
Cynthia Eagle Russett, *Sexual Science: The Victorian Construction of Womanhood*, Harvard University Press, Cambridge, Massachusetts, 1991

CHAPTER 7: FINDING PURPOSE

Mitch Albom, *Tuesdays with Morrie*, Doubleday, New York, 1997
Dale Carnegie, *How to Win Friends and Influence People*, Vermilion, London, 2007 (new edition)
Stephen R. Covey, *The 7 Habits of Highly Effective People*, Simon & Schuster, London, 2005
Holford, op. cit. (Chapter 4)
Greg Mortenson and David Oliver Relin, *Three Cups of Tea*, Penguin Books, London, 2008
Dr Dean Ornish, *Love and Survival*, Vermilion, London, 2001
Dr Norman Vincent Peale, *The Power of Positive Thinking*, Simon & Schuster, New York, 2003
Vaillant, op. cit. (Chapter 5)

CHAPTER 8: SEX

Dan Anderson and Maggie Berman, *Sex Tips for Straight Women from a Gay Man*, Thorsons, London, 2009
Blum, op.cit. (Chapter 2)
Brizendine, op.cit. (Chapter 1)
Alex Comfort, *The Joy of Sex*, Guild Publishing, London, 1972 (first edition)
Michael Gurian, *What Could He Be Thinking?*, HarperElement, London, 2009
Melissa Hines, *Brain Gender*, OUP USA, New York, 2005
Shere Hite, *The Hite Report: A Nationwide Study of Female Sexuality*, Seven Stories Press, New York, 2005
Hilda Hutcherson, *What Your Mother Never Told You About Sex*, Putnam, New York, 2004
Barbara Keesling, *Sexual Pleasure: Reaching New Heights of Sexual Arousal and Intimacy*, Hunter House, Alameda, California, 2006
Rachel P. Maines, *The Technology of Orgasm*, Johns Hopkins University Press, Baltimore, Maryland, 2001
William H. Masters and Virginia E. Johnson, *Human Sexual Response*, Little Brown, Boston, 1966 (first edition)
William H. Masters and Virginia E. Johnson, *Human Sexual Inadequacy*, Little Brown, Boston, 1970 (first edition)

Anne Moir and David Jessel, *Brain Sex*, Bantam Press, New York, 1980

Christiane Northrup, *The Secret Pleasures of Menopause*, Hay House UK, 2008

Gail Sheehy, *Sex and the Seasoned Woman*, Random House UK, 2006

CHAPTER 9: REDISCOVERING LOVE WITH YOUR ANDROPAUSAL MAN

Louis de Bernières, *Captain Corelli's Mandolin*, Secker & Warburg, London, 1994

Jed Diamond, *Male Menopause*, Sourcebooks, Naperville, Illinois, 1999

Jed Diamond, *Surviving Male Menopause*, Sourcebooks, Naperville, Illinois, 2001

Anne Taylor Fleming, *Marriage: A Duet*, Bloomsbury, London, 2004

Robert S. Tan, *The Andropause Mystery: Unraveling Truths About the Male Menopause*, Amred Publishing, Houston, Texas, 2009

CHAPTER 10: NEW RULES OF DATING FOR THE POST-MENOPAUSAL SINGLE WOMAN

Steven Carter, *Men Who Can't Love*, M. Evans, New York, 2003

Ellen Fein and Sherrie Schneider, *The Complete Book of Rules*, Thorsons, London, 2000

CHAPTER 11: PREPARING FOR SEPARATION AND DIVORCE

Sandra Blakeslee and Judith Wallerstein, *What About the Kids?; Raising your children before, during and after divorce*, Hyperion, New York, 2004

Mira Kirshenbaum, *Too Good to Leave, Too Bad to Stay: A Step-by-Step Guide to Help You Decide Whether to Stay in or Get Out of Your Relationship*, Michael Joseph, London, 1997

Musser, *Chambers Directory of the Legal Profession*, Chambers & Partners Publishing, London, 1999

Lee Raffel, *Should I Stay Or Go?: How Controlled Separation (CS) Can Save Your Marriage*, McGraw-Hill Contemporary, New York, 1999

Marianne Williamson, *A Return To Love*, Thorsons, London, 2009

CHAPTER 12: FACING UP TO LOSS

Joanne Cuthbertson and Susan Schevill, *Helping Your Child Sleep through the Night*, Bantam Books, New York, 1984

Norine Dresser and Fredda Wasserman, *Saying Goodbye to Someone You Love*, Demos Health, New York, 2010

Erin Tierney Kramp and Douglas H. Kramp, *Living with the End in Mind*, Three Rivers Press, New York, 1998

CHAPTER 13: FINANCE MATTERS

Michael Lewis, *The Big Short*, W.W. Norton, New York, 2010

Alvin Hall, *Your Money or Your Life: A Practical Guide to Solving Your Financial Problems and Affording a Life You'll Love*, Coronet, London, 2003

CHAPTER 14: GOING BACK TO WORK

Richard Nelson Bolles, *How to Find Your Mission in Life*, Ten Speed Press, Berkeley, California, 2005

Julia Cameron, *The Artist's Way: A Year of Creative Living*, Jeremy P. Tarcher/Penguin, New York, 2009

Carol Fishman Cohen and Vivian Steier Rabin, *Back on the Career Track*, Headline, London, 2007

Mireille Guiliano, *Women, Work and the Art of Savoir Faire*, Simon & Schuster, New York, 2009

Sylvia Ann Hewlett, *Off-Ramps and On-Ramps: Keeping Talented Women on the Road to Success*, Harvard Business School Press, Boston, Massachusetts, 2007

Herminia Ibarra, *Working Identity: Unconventional Strategies for Reinventing Your Career*, Harvard Business School Press, Boston, Massachusetts, 2003

Jane Jelenko and Susan Marshall, *Changing Lanes: Road Maps to Midlife Renewal*, Radom Press, Los Angeles, California, 2007

Jeri Sedlar and Rick Miners, *Don't Retire, Rewire!*, Jeremy P. Tarcher/Penguin, New York, 2008

Claire Shipman and Katty Kay, *Womenomics: Write Your Own Rules for Success*, Collins Business Books, London, 2009

Avivah Wittenberg-Cox and Alison Maitland, *Why Women Mean Business*, Wiley, Hoboken, New Jersey, 2009

CHAPTER 15: OLD IS THE NEW OLD

Simone de Beauvoir, *The Second Sex*, trans. H.M. Pashley, Cape, London, 1953 (first UK edition)

Betty Friedan, *The Feminine Mystique*, Norton, New York, 1963 (first edition)

Susie Orbach, *Fat Is a Feminist Issue*, Paddington Press, London, 1978 (first edition)

About the author

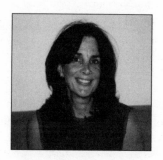

Jill Shaw Ruddock grew up in Baltimore, Maryland. She was educated in inner-city state schools before getting a degree in Politics from Bowdoin College (class of 1977) in Brunswick, Maine. She then moved to New York City and worked in advertising and, later, in publishing for *Inc.* magazine and *The Atlantic Monthly*.

In 1983, Jill moved to London to co-head the consulting firm of The Government Research Corporation. In 1985, she joined the US investment bank Alex Brown & Sons and became the Managing Director of their London office in 1994.

In 1999, she retired from finance and became involved in the theatre world, fundraising and sitting on the main boards of The Donmar Warehouse and The Mousetrap Theatre Projects. She was also a trustee of Bowdoin College for ten years.

Jill is married with two teenage daughters and lives in London.